Children

with

Hearing Loss

A Family Guide

•••••••••••••••••••••

David Luterman, D.Ed. Editor

DISCARD

Auricle Ink Publishers   *   Sedona Arizona

Library of Congress Cataloging-in-Publication Data

Children with hearing loss : a family guide / David Luterman, editor.--
1st ed.
       p. cm.
 Includes bibliographical references and index.
 ISBN 0-9661826-5-0 (soft cover)
 1. Deaf children. 2. Deaf children--Family relationships.
3. Hearing disorders in children. 4. Hearing impaired children--Rehabilitation.
I. Luterman, David.
 HV2391.C475 2006
 649'.1512--dc22

                                        2006002366

Copyright 2006
Auricle Ink Publishers
First Printing

ISBN: 0-9661826-5-0

Cover art and design by Brad Ingrao

Auricle Ink Publishers
P. O. Box 20607, Sedona AZ 86341
(928) 284-0860
www.hearingproblems.com

Table of Contents

Contributors

David Luterman, DEd
Professor Emeritus
Emerson College
120 Boylston St.
Boston, MA 02116

Linda Thibodeau, PhD
Associate Professor
Callier Center for Communication Disorders
The University of Texas at Dallas
1966 Inwood Road
Dallas, TX 75235

Karen Anderson, PhD
Audiology Consultant
Bureau of Early Intervention
4052 Bald Cypress Way, Bin A-06
Florida Department of Public Health
Tallahassee, FL 32399

Cheryl DeConde Johnson, EdD
Senior Consultant, Deaf/Hard of Hearing Disabilities
The Colorado Department of Education
Exceptional Student Services
201 E. Colfax Avenue
Denver, CO 80203

Introduction

Because of the rapid changes in the world of hearing loss, parents of children with a hearing loss need a reliable guide to maneuver through the technological and educational pitfalls. This book reflects the new reality facing parents today: early detection, sophisticated amplification whether by hearing aid or implant, and integrated school placement. Chapter 1 on the emotions of hearing loss and chapter 2 on the impact of hearing loss on the family are not much impacted by the new realities. The diagnosis of hearing loss will still have a profound emotional impact in most families and the entire family system will be affected. These chapters represent my forty years of working closely with families of newly diagnosed hearing-impaired children. While the technology has changed and the outlook for the child with a hearing loss is so much brighter, the impact that the diagnosis has on the emotional response and on many of the family dynamics has not changed.

Chapter 3 on hearing aids and cochlear implants will provide you with up-to-date information on current amplification technology for the child. It is written by Linda Thibodeau, PhD of the University of Texas. Since most hard-of-hearing children will currently be educated within an integrated school system, Chapter 4 provides information about the changes needed within the classroom to give a child with hearing loss maximum opportunity to succeed. Both school personnel and parents should be able to read this chapter with profit. It is written by Karen Anderson, PhD of the Florida Department of Public Health. Chapter 5 will provide you with information needed to negotiate the complex legislation supporting parental rights in the educational and diagnostic system. This chapter also provides information on resources. It is written by Cheryl DeConde Johnson, EdD, of the Colorado Department of Education.

With the advent of the new century, technology has created an axial change in education of the child with a hearing loss. Cochlear implants and neonatal screening have catapulted the child with a hearing loss into the auditory/verbal camp. The auditory-verbal approach teaches a child to use available aural information without encouraging a visual orientation.

Children are taught to listen and in extreme instances are actively discouraged from "looking." Because of both auditory-based therapy and the advancing technology, the difference between deaf and hard-of-hearing is rapidly blurring. Cochlear implants can now give many children (with a severe to profound loss) hearing that is in the mild to moderate category.

Previously we could not help these children with amplification because their loss was too severe. Coupled with early detection these "implanted" children function as hard-of-hearing. It is rapidly becoming feasible that deafness in a child will, in most cases, be a function of the choice of the parents or of poor clinical management.

We're now able to detect hearing loss in infants at birth and provide sophisticated amplification in the form of digital hearing aids. If these are not sufficient then the child is fitted with a cochlear implant. The current service model in many communities bypasses segregated schools for children with hearing loss entirely. Referrals from diagnostic centers are increasing for auditory/verbal therapists working in early intervention centers. The ultimate goal is to mainstream hard-of-hearing children in regular public schools. Schools for children with hearing loss are becoming increasingly repositories for—

- the deaf child of deaf parents who choose not to implant their children;
- the multiply handicapped;
- and the disadvantaged child with a hearing loss.

Advantaged hard-of-hearing children no matter how severe their loss are appearing in increasing numbers in public school programs. Many of these children have intelligible speech and grade-appropriate academic skills. It seems that if we can intelligently apply all that we currently know and use the available technology well, we have at hand all the necessary tools to mitigate the negative educational consequences of severe to profound hearing loss. This is an incredibly exciting time.

The technologies are in some respects a double-edge sword—they provide the means to get the children into a school with normal hearing children where they can be competitive. These children, however, despite their good speech and language skills, still have a hearing loss and there will be many instances during a school day when they will not respond like a normal hearing child. Many of them are also the only such child within their school and they often experience social isolation. We all need community and if the orally successful child cannot find it within the school context, he or she will seek it elsewhere. We must give these children with hearing loss in integrated settings roots within their social context.

Professionals and parents need to work together to provide support groups and social outlets for children who are integrating with normal hearing children. This will allow them to know they are not the only ones facing these challenges. Support from a child's peer group can often be the most important influence.

What of the future? It looks incredibly bright. Binaural implants are already here and fully implanted devices are coming shortly. I think we'll be implanting at increasingly younger ages and with children who are now classified as mildly to moderately hard-of-hearing. I think the surgery will be routine, as they are now doing on an outpatient basis in many surgical centers. It's possible and even likely that implants will become the dominant form of amplification for people with hearing loss. I think there will still be small pockets of the culturally deaf who will be on the margins. Until we get the mainstreaming model fully operational we will go through periodic cycles whereby the deaf community and the romance of sign language is rediscovered by adolescents with hearing loss. I think some time in this century we will have a cure for sensorineural deafness. I have faith that stem cell research will ultimately be able to regrow damaged hair cells.

Despite all our current challenges, I think this is a wonderful time to have been professionally active in early childhood hearing loss. We professionals have seen us move from bleak prognosis to hopeful outcomes, from restricted vocational opportunities to almost unlimited ones, from poor academic skills to grade-appropriate, and from unintelligible speech to normal or near-normal speech intelligibility. I think congenitally hard-of-hearing children will have the choice of being included both within the cultural mainstream and the hard-of-hearing community. Hopefully, they will be able to move seamlessly between both worlds. The contributors and I feel privileged to have been a part of this true revolution and blessed to be living in such interesting times.

Chapter 1

The Emotional Impact of Hearing Loss

David Luterman, D. Ed.

Dr. Luterman wishes to acknowledge the many sources who helped in preparation of this book, including the obvious collaborators Karen Anderson, Cheryl de Conde Johnson, Linda Thibodeau, and at Auricle Ink Publishers Richard and Jo Carmen. In addition, son Dan was the computer maven, friends Mark Ross and Lynn Connors were excellent advisors, Librarian Liz Besara was an immense help searching literature, and his wife Leonie who on so many fronts made this book possible.

Trained as an audiologist, Dr. Luterman realized that there was a serious gap in service delivery to newly diagnosed children with a hearing loss and their families, namely that parents were not given the clinical attention that they needed. In 1965, he started a family-centered nursery which is functioning to this day. He serves as its Director and facilitates the parent support group.

Dr. Luterman is Professor Emeritus at Emerson College in Boston and Director of the Thayer Lindsey Family Centered Nursery for Hearing Impaired Children. He has dedicated his career to developing a greater understanding of the psychological effects and emotions associated with hearing loss and the caregiver role. He teaches professionals to understand the emotional responses of parents as they come to grips with the hearing loss of their child. He has lectured extensively on counseling throughout the United States, Canada and abroad, and has authored a number of books on the subject matter of hearing loss in children.

I often tell parents who have recently completed the diagnostic process that you have the same child you went into the testing booth with—it's just that you're looking at him/her differently now. By this I mean that the "problem" at this time is the parents' problem, not the child's. For the parents, it's a grief reaction: they've lost the child they thought they were going to have and the life they expected to live. This will invoke for the parents many feelings of loss. For the child, there will be feelings associated with the hearing loss, but these will not be one of loss as almost all children with hearing loss have never heard normally or have no memory of hearing. These children have little or no concept of what they've lost.

In the past, I've compared the parental loss to a death, but I have begun to see that this is no longer accurate. In a death, there's finality to the grief, there's a burial and life can go on, albeit with pain and loss. With hearing loss the grief is chronic, lived with 24/7. The child is a constant reminder to the parents of this loss. No matter how well adjusted the parents seem to be to the reality that their child has a hearing loss, there will be trigger events that remind them of the loss and those initial feelings of pain and sorrow return. Triggers can be as simple as a birthday party or the anniversary of their original diagnostic evaluation. What seems to happen after the initial pain of the diagnosis is that parents learn to live in a bubble of "normal" hearing loss and adjust to the disability of their child by not thinking about it. The trigger events remind them just how abnormal their life really is and what they've lost.

Newborn Screening

With the advent of newborn screening the diagnosis of hearing loss is, in most cases, going to be before the child is three months of age. The very early diagnosis seems to be a mixed blessing. In a recent study we conducted at Emerson College (Luterman and Kurtzer-White, 1999), parents of children with hearing loss were asked if they would have liked to know at birth if their child had a hearing loss. The majority answered "yes" (83%) and gave some of the following reasons:

- We could have offered earlier amplification or sign language, instead of silently moving mouths;
- Because I would have had more time to give the very important communication she missed for two years;
- Only because of a better understanding.

Those parents who said "no" (17%), they would not have liked to know their child was hard-of-hearing, gave the following reasons:

- I guess I was glad that I knew at 2 days so we could get started on what we needed to do, but I missed having the bonding time;
- Parents need to bond with the infant before getting swept up in the issues of hearing impairment;
- Not knowing immediately gave us (Mom and child) a time to bond normally, but I'm also thankful to have found out before 6 months;
- She was too sick. Knowing at birth would have been too depressing.

My experience with parents is that those who found out that their child had hearing loss at birth are grateful that they found out so early, but regret that they didn't have time to enjoy their baby. They had to hit the ground running and couldn't delight in their newborn. It seems to take a while for the early diagnosed parents to recognize their loss. At first, gratitude for the early start dominates their thinking. It's only when they have time to reflect that they realize what they've lost.

Parents with a later diagnosis often felt guilty that they had taken so long to get started and did not always appreciate the time spent thinking of their child as normal hearing. They think of this as wasted time. I often assure them that they got a great gift in that they had this time to enjoy their child. The consensus among parents is that the most desirable time to have found out that their child had a hearing loss was after three months and before six months. Unfortunately, most screening programs are not designed to detect hearing loss after three months of age because of the difficulty of locating parents of newborns after they leave the hospital and the expense of setting up equipment in every pediatrician's office. Much training and effort needs to be continuously expended to provide audiologists and hospital personnel with not only the technical skills to diagnose hearing loss in very young infants, but also to develop the skills to support the parents at an emotionally vulnerable time.

Stages of Diagnosis

The feelings experienced in the early stages of diagnosis are quite intense, and the emotional response to the child's hearing loss is independent of the degree of loss. The disability is never in the audiogram, it's in the perception of the parents. Parents of children with mild hearing loss seldom appreciate being told that they are lucky their child can hear so much. For them it's still a loss for which they have a right to grieve. In fact, research has shown (Yoshinaga-Itano and Abdala de Uzcategui, 2001) that parents of children with mild to moderate losses are more stressed than parents of children with severe to profound losses. Parents of children with mild to moderate losses have more decisions to make regarding school placement and many of these children are on the cusp of needing a cochlear implant. Outcomes and decisions for these children are more ambiguous than for children with more severe losses. Also the mildly impaired child has potentially more hearing to lose and parents often live with the constant fear of a further increase in the hearing loss.

At the time of diagnosis a host of uncomfortable feelings usually emerge, among them fear, inadequacy, anger, guilt, vulnerability and confusion. Underlying all this for hearing parents is the profound feeling of loss. The pain of this loss never quite goes away, as one father of a fifteen year old said: "When you first find out your child is hard-of-hearing, it really hurts and then it becomes a dull ache that never goes away."

All the feelings described in this chapter are appropriate to life's situation: the feelings just are— they need to be listened to, validated and not judged. Behavior has consequences that can be evaluated so parents need not be responsible for how they feel but always and only for how they behave.

Anger

Anger is generally pervasive and has several sources. Parents often feel cheated: "This isn't supposed to happen" or "Why me?" A frequent cause of anger is generated by a violation of expectations. Parents expect to have a normal hearing child, as every one else they know does, and when this is violated, they can become angry. As one mother ruefully noted, "The odds on having a hard-of-hearing child are one in a thousand but when you're the statistic the odds don't matter."

Anger is also a result of a loss of control in our lives. We like to think we can always behave in a way that's in our own best interest. To have a child with hearing loss is restrictive—the angry parent who could not accept a promotion because to do so would mean that the child would not have a suitable educational program, has lost some degree of freedom. This restriction causes anger. There is also the anger borne of helplessness when a child in the family is hurting and the parent cannot do something to make it better.

There is also a great deal of anger that masks fear, whenever our basic security is threatened. Our brains are wired in such a way that the anger response has the most survival possibilities. We are mobilized for fight or flight (that is, denial or unacceptable diagnosis) and the adrenalin flows. This response is activated very easily at the time of diagnosis because the diagnosis involves a profound change in the parent's life plan, so that basic security is threatened. The parental fears are around their feelings of adequacy to cope with the new reality and the world of disability they have suddenly and unwillingly been thrust into.

Anger is seldom dealt with effectively in families because it threatens the cohesion of the family system. Children are frequently taught that anger and the expression of anger is "not nice" and they tend to carry this notion into adulthood. Anger that is not expressed very often becomes depression. When we sit on our feelings we suppress all of them and lose our joy as well. Unexpressed anger frequently becomes displaced and innocent victims, spouses and children often get in the line of fire of the misplaced anger. Professionals are also innocent recipients of parental ire. The angry parent often strikes fear in the heart of many professionals. I for one see anger when it is identified accurately and channeled appropriately as a marvelous energy for change. Angry people are the ones who become "change agents," usually for the better. They become passionate advocates for their child and ultimately for all children with hearing loss.

Guilt

Guilt is another emotion that is highly prevalent in parents of children with hearing loss. Maternal guilt is usually around the cause of the hearing loss. Mothers in many families feel they have the responsibility for maintaining the health of the children and when one is ill, the mother feels that she has failed in some way. Women also have the awesome responsibility of carrying the fetus for nine months and when a child is born with a hearing loss, mothers often feel they must have done something wrong in their pregnancy to have caused their child's hearing problem. Mothers often try to recall the pregnancy day by day, sometimes hour by hour, to find something that can be blamed for the hearing loss. In nine months it is almost impossible not to find something amiss; thus is born "the guilty secret:"

- I smoked and drank the first few months before I knew I was pregnant;
- I rushed to catch the bus and caused an early labor;
- I was so upset at my mother's illness the stress caused the hearing loss.

If the mother cannot find "the cause" in pregnancy, she may try to find it in her life:

- I tried drugs in high school;
- I was not nice to my hard-of-hearing sister and God is now punishing me.

A father's guilt is seldom related to cause, but is related to the pain experienced by his spouse and family. Men often have the protector role and when someone in the family is hurting, the father feels he has failed. The father is generally the one to offer solutions. When they don't solve the problem, he feels guilty that he somehow has let the family down. This is why fathers are often not good listeners because they feel the need to "fix" things and unfortunately early childhood hearing loss does not lend itself to fixing. The feeling of helplessness in the face of an unfixable problem often leads to anger.

Guilt unrecognized and unacknowledged leads to the super-dedicated and/or overprotective parent. The super-dedicated parent says: "I let something bad happen to you and now I'm going to make it up to you;" the overprotective parent says: "I was remiss in letting something bad happen to you and I'm not about to let anything else bad happen." Both of these paths can lead to unhealthy consequences for the child and the family. Super dedication leads to an unbalancing of the family system. Over time hearing siblings are often adversely affected by the lack of attention, and marriages are often at risk because too much energy has gone into the parenting and not enough into the marriage.

Identity Crisis

When parents need to let go of their adolescent child, they're frequently unable to do so because they've defined themselves for so many years as the parent of a child with hearing loss. They have an identity crisis. "If I am not the parent of a child with a hearing loss, who am I?" This becomes a difficult question for super-dedicated parents to answer. A parent's role is to facilitate the child's passage into adulthood. The "letting go" is an important part of the process. In order to do this, parents must maintain suitable boundaries so that their day doesn't rise and fall with their child's day. It's important for parents to process their feelings of guilt, inadequacy and anger so that they can establish appropriate boundaries. This will also help the child to feel more self-confident in life.

All parents need to keep some energy for the marriage, their other children, and for their own personal growth. When they fail to do so, the letting go process is much harder because there doesn't seem anywhere positive to go. The proactive parents who have taken care of their own needs and who've raised their children successfully to go out into the world are happy and supportive of their child's leaving the nest.

Overprotection

Overprotection is detrimental to the child as well. One of the hardest tasks of parenting is to let your child fail. Through failure, the child develops the skills to meet adversity as an adult. Because the parents are compensating for a perceived failure on their part to protect their child, they are often unwilling to risk the child having another negative experience because that would indicate they were remiss again. Thus, the child experiences minimum failure and seldom has to take responsibility for the consequences of his/her behavior. This becomes crippling as an adult. To the child, the overprotection can be seen as a statement that he or she is incapable of managing on their own because the world is too dangerous and the child is too incompetent to make good decisions.

Children who have grown to adulthood in such a scenario become fearful and self-limiting. They don't "risk" and are unable to accept responsibility for their actions. If you're always blaming others for your failures, then there's no impetus to change and thus growth is limited. This was borne out to me once when I was giving a lecture in which a sign language interpreter was standing behind me interpreting my words. A man complained bitterly at the end of the talk that he missed the whole lecture because the interpreter was positioned in such a way that he couldn't see her signs. I thought, with a sense of despair, that nobody had taught him to take responsibility for himself. If he had he'd have changed his seat or said something at the outset so he would not have missed the lecture. Instead he took no responsibility for his actions preferring to miss the lecture and complain. Unfortunately, there are too many graduates of programs for the hearing impaired who are like him.

All parents, at some level, when they're willing to be introspective about the parenting process, recognize the awesome responsibility that raising a child to adulthood is. So, they "run scared." When the child is diagnosed with a hearing loss, all of the existing parental feelings of inadequacy are amplified tenfold. Now parents feel that they have to be super parents in order to raise the child with hearing loss through to responsible adulthood. It is an overwhelming task and one in which they have no preparation. Out of the parental feelings of inadequacy parents often turn to the professionals to take on the responsibility of managing the child. They're seeking a savior. Unfortunately, there are too many professionals who are willing to take on the savior role, usually to the long-term detriment of the family. A savior comes at the expense of the parent's self-esteem and the child's independence.

Confusion

Confusion is another emotional component for the hearing parents of a child with hearing loss. Most parents have no experience of hearing loss, the vocabulary is new, the controversies are many, and the advocates are passionate. The parents are bombarded with information, much of it conflicting, at a time when they're in emotional turmoil and least able to mentally process information. Information comes from all sources. Parents have lost their anonymity. Passersby and casual acquaintances notice the hearing aids and will offer inspirational stories or ask intrusive questions. Professionals sometimes give information when parents are not emotionally prepared to receive it. This leads to confusion and contributes to the parents feeling overwhelmed and inadequate.

Vulnerability and Existential Crises

Parents of children with hearing loss also feel their own vulnerability. We are all defenseless to tragic occurrences in our lives. This existential truth is very difficult to deal with in our everyday living, so in order to protect ourselves from this fact, we practice denial. Most of us live in our own personal bubble of denial, sure that bad things happen only to other people. Having a child with hearing loss pierces that bubble, and parents must confront the truth of their vulnerability. Confronting our vulnerability can lead to being fearful and can contribute to the overprotection of the child. The child is seen as fragile and exposed. The parent often feels that: "I just want to wrap him/her up in cotton wool and hide him/her away and not let any bad things happen again."

On the surface, parents undergoing the existential crises will look like the overprotective guilt-driven parent. These parents, however, will be asking the "why me?" question and will be undergoing a crises of meaning. The traditional "Judeo-Christian" view of the world is that God punishes the wicked and rewards the good. If that's true, then why did they have a child with a hearing problem?; either they were bad or God is absent. Either view is hard to take and requires a great deal of soul searching. Without an effective answer it can leave parents mired in bitterness.

The existential crises of vulnerability can have very positive effects if parents are allowed to work through the issues. The truth of the matter is we are all vulnerable and always have been. When we can incorporate this notion into our everyday life, we live more authentically by taking nothing for granted and recognizing the time-limited nature of our lives. We appreciate what we have and want to get the most out of our experiences. We do not want to waste time. Parents often can find new meaning and purpose in their lives. One mother, for example, was elected to her town's school board. As a member of the committee she helped set up programs for children with disabilities within the school system, helping her daughter and also many other children in her community. This same mother commented, "I would have been content to be a suburban housewife worrying about whether my house was clean. I now recognize how much I've grown and how much better I feel about myself as a result of my daughter's hearing loss. I wish it was some other way."

I frequently tell parents that hearing loss is a powerful teacher and if we listen to it, it can lead us on a path of joy and a better life, although the path is strewn with pain and hard work. It seems we must all pay our dues in order to get to a truly joyful place.

Parents will most often respond to the hearing loss in accordance with their own life experience and disposition. Parents who have met adversity early in life often have the personal resources to make a rapid adjustment to their child's hearing loss no matter how severe it is, while other parents, who are not used to dealing with adversity, can be devastated by having a child with a mild hearing loss. In one parent group I was working with, a mother wailed about her child's mild hearing loss, commenting that she had a perfect childhood and this was the first bad thing that ever happened to her. My response to her was that her childhood was not so perfect if she had never been exposed to adversity. She never did come to accept her child's hearing loss, remaining stuck in "Why me?" She had not learned how to work productively with the early childhood staff and with her child.

Isolation

An overriding feeling that parents often have is one of isolation. The experience of having a child with hearing loss alienates parents from their community. They are usually the only one in their everyday life

coping with this problem. Friends and relatives con-
spire to try to make them feel better usually by saying
it could be worse or offering hope in the way of a cure.
Many have inspirational stories. None of this is helpful
on a long-term basis because it denies the parent's
reality: the parents have experienced a loss and nothing can take the pain of that loss away. Telling parents
that "They shouldn't feel that way" no matter how nice-
ly put, only serves to have them feel guilty that they're
feeling that way.

In one parent group I was beginning to facilitate,
a mother looked at me and said, "You're going to make
me cry." I said, "No. I'm going to give you permission
to cry," whereupon she started to cry. Because few
people give parents permission to cry, they don't share
their feelings with friends and extended family, and feel
cut off from any support. A helping professional can
provide some emotional support, but the most help
can come from other parents of children with hearing
loss who can provide the validation of the experience
of life change that parents undergo when their child is
diagnosed. In these family-to-family support relationships the parents can recognize how typical their experience is.

In the Emerson study (Luterman and Kurtzer-
White, 1999), parents rated meeting other parents as
their Number One need at the time of diagnosis. The
Number Two rated need was help with their feelings.
Number Three was getting started with intervention
services. A good early intervention program needs to
provide all three elements and a support group needs
to be a vital component.

Coping with loss is a complex process. While
there have been a number of models over many
years, Matson and Brooks (1977) looked at chronic
illness and proposed a coping model that is useful.
They proposed denial, resistance, affirmation and
integration.

Denial

Denial is an emotion-based coping mechanism that occurs whenever we feel so psychologically over-whelmed by a situation that the only way to cope is to block it out. There's no emotional "owning" of the problem. Real denial is so successful that we actually cannot see the problem. Denial is an unconscious process. Parents who admit their child has a hearing loss are not in denial. When denial is present, parents will act as though the child has normal hearing.

In the early stages of diagnosis, I'm optimistic about outcomes for parents who grieve openly because they emotionally own the situation. On the other hand, parents who seem to be "taking it so well" are often buttressed by denial and it sometimes takes them a long time to come to grips with their child's hearing loss. I remember one mother of a newly diagnosed child telling me through her tears that she was "doing this badly." I assured her she was doing it just right. Her child has been very successful.

Resistance

Denial blends into resistance and is sometimes indistinguishable from it. When the initial acute pain subsides, parents will often feel that they're a "special case" and all of the predictions and experiences of others will not apply to them. Resistance differs from denial in that people acknowledge to themselves they have a problem, but are going to defeat it. Parents will say (often at 3 a.m.), "I know he has a hearing loss, but he's going to defy all the predictions! No one will be able to identify him as having a hearing loss because his speech will be normal and he'll be able to lipread everything."

In resistance, parents are loathe to tell anyone that their child has a hearing problem—they are in the "closet." They are also reluctant to join parent groups because they're "not like everyone else." Their sense of self is tied up in their child as they ponder: "What will others think of us because our child has a problem." A dilemma for parents in resistance arises when they take a photo of their child and they're not sure whether or not to leave the hearings aids on or off. Thus, parents in resistance seldom take pictures of their child wearing hearing aids. The resistant father seldom tells his coworkers that he has a child with hearing loss.

Affirmation

In affirmation the loss is acknowledged to both self and the world. Affirmation is a statement that, "I'm different and my family is different from others in my community and I'm becoming comfortable with that." It's assuming a new identity. Unlike resistance, the affirming family commonly photographs the child with hearing aids. During this stage of coping the family is consumed with the disorder and they almost sleep, eat and breathe hearing loss. Families often become active in organizations and are eager to educate others. Most of the family's energy is devoted to helping the child with hearing loss. In this stage, there's often an intense desire to help others. As one mother observed, "At first you feel badly for yourself then you feel badly for your child, and then you feel badly for all children with disabilities."

Integration (also known as Acceptance)

Integration is characterized by putting the disorder into a life prospective. At this time, parents learn to live with the hearing loss and recognize that "beating" hearing loss is not a matter of attaining normal hearing, but in the ability to live life to the fullest. But there's still pain and at times active grief, especially around "trigger" events. Parents at this stage also can be thrown back into denial and resistance by a big trigger event, such as a child not succeeding in the regular classroom and needing to be put into a special education class. Parents may need considerable time integrating this change into their life style. This is why it's not helpful to categorize any family into a particular stage since it's always fluid, depending in large measure on how well the child is meeting parental expectations.

One mother commented, "I've begun to realize that I would have a good day when my son had a good one and a bad day when he had a bad one. I now realize that I can have a good day even when he has a bad one. It took me a long time to get here."

I think when parents can say this they've reached the integration stage. My experience is that once a family has achieved a level of acceptance, their ability to adjust to new realities is a good deal healthier than when the hearing loss was first diagnosed. Families who successfully make it to this stage have usually taken advantage of support groups for themselves, their child and any other siblings. Everyone in the family is vulnerable to feelings of "mourning" and they all need help dealing with their particular issues.

With help, the feelings associated with loss can be transmuted into productive behavior. The confusion becomes a spur to learning, the recognition of vulnerability leads to a re-ordering of priorities, anger becomes the energy to make changes, and guilt transforms into commitment. The grief transmutes to compassion for all suffering, but in particular for those parents and children dealing with disabilities. The feelings recur as trigger events unfold but they're never as intense as they were in the early stages of diagnosis. What the parents need most in the early stages, is someone who will listen compassionately and deeply to their feelings and not prescribe solutions. Information needs to be given judiciously when parents are receptive to receiving it. They need emotional support in a safe, nonjudgmental relationship that

enables them to work out their own solutions for themselves and their families. They need empathy and
never sympathy. It's important not to view early childhood hearing loss as a tragedy but as a powerful
teacher, and if you allow the process to happen, this
will promote growth for both you and the child.

The Child's Emotions

The child with hearing loss does not experience
the loss of hearing as a "loss" since the child has never
heard normally. For the child of hearing parents, the
loss becomes a source of alienation since it separates
the child from the parents and siblings. Usually no later
the around age four or five, the child begins to notice
that he or she is the only one in the family wearing
hearing aids and this difference is usually noted without any connotation of good or bad. It is usually not
until the child enters a school with children who hear
normally that the hearing loss becomes a negative in
the child's mind. The loss of hearing sets the child
apart from peers in an undesirable way. The speech of
the child with hearing loss may be different, and their
needs considered "special," all of which serve to signal
to the child that he or she does not belong with everyone else and also that he or she is deficient. At this
point, the healthy child's self-esteem can become
damaged. The feeling is "I am defective, I am not
okay." Parents will then begin to get the dreaded questions: "What's the matter with me?" or "Why am I different?"

At first, the child is usually just seeking facts,
but parents tend to hear this as: "What did you do to
cause me to have a hearing loss?" This often activates
parental feelings of guilt. The question needs to be
answered in a matter of fact way and parents can ask
in turn: "Do you think it's bad to have a hearing loss?"
Children need to be given a chance to talk about their
feelings and the culture of talking about feelings needs

to be part of the family in order to promote healthy emotional growth for the child. The initial question of why am I different is usually prompted by a negative interaction with a hearing peer. For children whose family is still struggling with denial or resistance, this becomes an even worse blow to their already fragile self-esteem. Some children may react by acting out in anger while others withdraw into depression. In either case, the child and the family can benefit from professional help to guide them to a healthier place.

Parents of hard-of-hearing children are often reluctant to cry in their presence for fear of upsetting them. Nevertheless, almost all children with hearing loss know that their parents are sad because of the hearing loss. At this age it's natural for all children to assume they're the cause for any upset in the family, and unfortunately, many children feel guilty that they have caused their parents pain. What parents need to make clear to the child is that they're sad about the hearing loss, which neither one of them had any control over, and not about the child. This is a difficult concept to get across to the child since the hearing loss is such a dominant feature of his or her life. Nevertheless, it is only a feature and is not an issue about the child. If the parents are in denial, the child feels that he or she must bear the weight of the parent's expectations. Often, these are unrealistic, such as the hearing loss will be overcome, the child will speak normally, and in most respects be the child they were supposed to have. This is an unrealistic situation for the child, who can feel that there's no way to gain the love and approval of their parents. Many children with hearing loss feel that they have somehow failed their parents. The damage this does to a child is monumental. It can become a pervasive theme in their lives.

Professional Evaluation and Academic Success

Success for the child is often elusive. Professionals tend to measure it in terms of speech, language and academic achievement—all measurable skills. Parents are similarly concerned about academic achievement, but they also tend to see success in terms of the happiness of the child. Happiness is something that is difficult to measure since it is compounded of many different elements. The degree of the child's hearing loss is not an important component of his or her happiness nor at this juncture in our clinical management is it an important predictor of academic success. Children with severe to profound hearing loss are now being identified early and are using cochlear implants by one year of age. Many of them now function as hard-of-hearing children who are using hearing aids so that it's not possible now to predict academic success on the basis of the child's audiogram.

Schlessinger (1992) conducted one of the few longitudinal studies in education of children with hearing loss. She studied forty families for twenty years to determine the factors that were most relevant to academic success. She found that the best predictor of academic success was the self-esteem of the mother. This was more important than degree of hearing loss, socio-economic status and educational methodology. A mother with high self-esteem will find the best means of getting language to the child and will ensure that the educational program is providing optimum service and support.

The overriding problem for children with hearing loss educated in regular classrooms is in the social and emotional realm. Many of these children, because of their early start and superior amplification are doing well academically but are not necessarily happy socially. One mother of a thirteen-year-old noting his social isolation wished for nothing more than two or three hard-of-hearing teenagers to move into town to main-stream with her son. To address these social, emotion-al, and self-esteem needs we ultimately may need clusters of regular classes of children with hearing loss in one or more schools rather than isolating children as the only one in their home schools.

Generally, I recommend to parents that the child with hearing loss be one of the oldest in the class so that he or she has more physical skills than the normal hearing children and that some emphasis be put in a skill area. We have found that children who are edu-cated in the regular classroom most successfully are those who have a particular skill that is valued by their class peers. For example, one successfully integrated child was very good in chess and found his own group of children interested in chess that he could relate to. Another child was excellent in soccer and she also had her own peer group. Both of these sets of parents also spent considerable time transporting their children to meet with other children who have a hearing loss.

To best describe the problems of integrating a child with hearing loss into a school with normal hear-ing children, I asked an eighteen-year-old graduate of our nursery program, who we'll call Maureen, to write me about her experience. Below are excerpts from her letter:

Looking at the person I am today, I truly believe that placing me in a mainstreamed learning environ-ment was one of the best decisions my parents made for me. Being in such an environment was so difficult that I believe I subconsciously forgot all my bad expe-riences. What I do remember of my elementary and middle school years is the strong feeling of isolation, especially as I was always the only hard-of-hearing student in my school. Having said that, I do appreciate the individualized attention I received from my teach-ers during my early years, which allowed me to suc-ceed academically.

Throughout my school years I consistently made efforts to sit in the front of the classroom and meet with my teachers for one-on-one sessions to clear up misunderstandings or for extra help. During elementary school my teachers and parents were more tuned into what was going on in my school life, both academically and socially.

While I was able to succeed academically, I struggled in social settings. My hearing impairment was initially "cool" in the sense that I had something that the rest of my peers did not, but the novelty would always wear off. Even though I would make presentations at the beginning of each school year about my hearing loss, complete with a "show and tell" of my hearing aids, as well as suggestions on how to interact with me (i.e., face me while talking, please repeat something for me if I don't understand,) my peers were not particularly willing to accommodate my needs. My peers would become extremely irritated at having to repeat things for me and many would end up walking off with a "never mind!" attitude leaving me angry and frustrated. This contributed to the growing sense of isolation I felt and perhaps it is for this very reason that books became my best friends. I had no real friends to socialize with.

The pattern continued in middle school, except the situation only worsened. For one, I had a harder time academically because I had moved from a school where my entire class was 42 students to one that was anywhere from 200-400 students. As a result, classes were noisier and I had to make a bigger effort to seek out my teachers for extra help or meetings to clarify missed information. While this required more effort, I do feel that I was able to form closer relationships with my teachers, perhaps because for the first time I was monitoring my own progress and became more assertive about my needs. Through all this, my parents still played an active role in communicating with my teachers.

Although I flourished academically, my social life was horrible. My hearing loss ended up becoming a huge issue, especially since I found my peers to be less receptive and even antagonistic toward my hearing impairment. This created many issues for me socially, as they were unwilling to assist me when I needed it, especially as I slowly began to adjust to the extremely noisy lunchrooms and hallways, and even noisier classrooms. They would make half-hearted attempts to face me while talking or to repeat what was being said. As a result, I felt excluded much more so than in elementary school. During these three years, my family members were my best friends.

My best years by far were my high school years. For once, I flourished in all ways—ways I hadn't imagined possible: academically and socially. In high school, I was once again in a much smaller environment about 280 students). This was a turning point in my life, not only because I was in the most positive learning environment I had been in, but because I received my cochlear implant during the beginning of my freshman year. The support I received from my teachers, peers and the rest of the school community was astounding. Listening with the cochlear implant improved my life dramatically. I could hear much more than I did with my hearing aids, and noisy situations became much easier to handle. That in itself boosted my confidence and made me more self-assured.

The biggest change in my academic life, however, was that by the middle of my sophomore year I had completely taken over the responsibility of communicating with my teachers. My parents were only as involved with my teachers as I wanted them to be. I coordinated everything I needed, focused on maintaining my grades and my success in the classroom. I would make sure that I was positioned in such a way that I could effectively follow and participate in class discussions and copied other students' notes when I felt I missed out on large parts of the discussions and lectures.

Socially, high school offered me opportunities I never had. My circle of friends were the ones I turned to when I needed to be clued into what the speaker was saying at assemblies or during announcements. They were the ones who provided me with the support during the early months with my cochlear implant. In the end, I was not defined by the fact that I could not hear, but rather, by the person I was.

Presentation of Maureen's thoughts alone does not reveal the whole picture. Her Mother subsequently wrote me as well. Here are some excerpts from that letter:

The time is opportune to write about Maureen's experiences in mainstreaming, as she embarks on her college career.

As far as academics go, I don't think we could have been luckier. The combination of Maureen's dogged motivation and tenacity, her teachers and our monitoring, made her very successful. By the time she was in kindergarten we were paying for all the extra help she needed, essentially a speech therapist and a teacher of the deaf (tutor) outside the classroom. The three-way interaction—school, special teachers and parents—worked very well in every setting.

When she started middle school she had an IEP (Individual Education Program) and a county-provided teacher of the deaf whom she weaned off by 7th grade. After that we only had the teacher see her to keep contact with the special education bureaucracy (and as a safety net, in case something went wrong). The biggest challenge, which came to a head in middle school, was social. She was often isolated, lonely, socially awkward and lacking friends. There were times when I waited outside her middle school building glaring at all the kids who came out, daring them to be "mean" to her, and then whisking her off in the car so she would not have to endure the taunts. At that time if someone had told me this would make her stronger, I would have said, "I'm happy to have her weak!!" I think middle school is a time where bullying gets so much more sophisticated and more hurtful.

Maureen received her cochlear implant in the summer before she started ninth grade. She went to a private school with very small classes and the most fabulous set of teachers. We had to do no monitoring at all, as Maureen took it over completely.

The most important part of her development has been her emotional strength, self-esteem and security. Her individual relationships with her family, both immediate and extended, have been instrumental in helping her establish these important milestones.

As a parent, the most difficult part of her growing up was to witness this isolation and have to compensate for it by trying to be her friend as well as a parent. Of course, as she embarks on college, this could be seen as a blessing, as we have a daughter who is still our friend, who escaped much of the other angst of adolescence, who relied on us for much of her social information, and yet who today has some of the most steadfast friends she acquired during high school. Her relationships with adults around her have always given her great succor and confidence and this happened because she sought them out. Therefore, in retrospect, all's well that ends well.

Summary

As is evident from Maureen's account, it was her high self-esteem, assertiveness and her family's great support that got her through academically. At the same time, they probably also led to some of her social difficulties. Self-advocacy based on the child's high self-esteem is a necessary component of the successful integration of a child with hearing loss. The assertiveness can sometimes alienate the children with normal hearing and sometimes teachers, but it's a necessary component for success.

The compliant child who feigns understanding in classes usually comes up short at examination times. Schools that give these children social promotions are not helpful because they only defer the problem to a later time when the deficits in academics are usually much larger and therefore harder to fix. Maureen's mother monitored her education and in this case the strong family ties compensated for the lack of friends in elementary and middle school.

Fortunately by high school Maureen's family finally found a school program that was fully supportive and a peer group that was helpful so that she could flourish. I think children with hearing loss are going to need these small supportive classrooms in order to succeed both academically and socially. Unfortunately, they're in short supply in public schools.

Parents always need to consider the possibility that their child may be more academically and/or socially successful in a specialized school or class. Some children, despite having all the necessary support, do not do well when educated in a regular classroom and will need specialized instruction. This is usually a painful decision for hearing parents to make as it means giving up the dream of having that normal hearing child who goes to the local school. Placement in a cluster school, a self-contained class or a segregated school is very often seen as a failure. To my mind, any school placement is an experiment to see how well a child can do—healthy or impaired. If the child is not succeeding, then it's the parents' responsibility to make changes. The mistake I've seen parents make over the years is not that they've chosen a program that didn't work out, but they've stayed too long with an unsuccessful program that they were reluctant to change because of their own needs or their fear of alienating the professionals. As parents, we don't owe our children the responsibility to be "right" all the time. We do owe them the responsibility to change a decision when we see that it's not working. To this end we must constantly monitor the child's education and be prepared to make changes when necessary.

All of the attendant feelings of the difficult job of growing up are present in the child with hearing loss. The insecurities, the angers, the pain are all there, and compounding these is the issue of isolation and alienation. Children with hearing loss need to find a supportive community. At first it needs to be the home, and hopefully the school, and finally a work and social community. Learning how to function in the mainstream is important, but having a community of your peers is what staves off the isolation.

As with all children, those with hearing loss need to be listened to, empathized with and validated. Unfortunately, there's no blueprint or manual for successfully raising a child, let alone one with hearing loss. Very often parents have to fly by the seat of their pants. Children have a remarkable capacity to challenge parents whether they can hear or not. In these challenges lay growth. We give to life what life demands and when we're stressed we're forced to find capacities that would otherwise lie dormant. The child with a hearing loss forces parents to guide their child with intention—nothing is taken for granted. The joys are many and the pain intense. I often tell parents this child has guaranteed you an interesting life. Despite the many difficulties, I have seen in over forty years of active participation with families, so many of these children turn out so well. This is a testament, I think, to the care of the parents and the strength of the children. Hearing loss is truly a teacher.

References

Luterman, D and Kurtzer-White, E. (1999). Identifying Hearing Loss: Parent's Needs. Journal of Audiology 8, 8-13.

Matson D and Brooks L. (1977). Adjusting to Multiple Sclerosis, An Exploratory Study. Journal of Social Science and Medicine 11, 245-250.

Schlessinger, H. (1992). The Elusive X Factor: Parental Contributions to Literacy. In: *A Free Hand,* M. Walworth, D. Moores, T. O'Rourke (Eds.). Silver Springs, MD: TJ Publishers.

Yoshinaga-Itano, C. and Abdala de Uzcategui, C. (2001). Early Identification and Social Emotional Factors of Children with Hearing Loss and Children Screened for Hearing Loss. In: *Early Childhood Deafness*, Kurtzer-White and Luterman (Eds.), Baltimore, MD: York Press.

Chapter 2

Hearing Loss and the Family

David Luterman, D. Ed.

Family therapists tell us that the family is a system in which all of the parts are interconnected (Minuchin, 1974). This means that if one part of the system is not functioning well, it affects all of the other parts; even seemingly, remote ones. When a child is diagnosed with a hearing loss, then we have an entire family system with a hearing problem. This is a difficult concept to grasp; many professionals fail to do so, because of a lack of training in family dynamics. It is the inclination of everyone involved to try to "fix" the defective part, (i.e. the hearing of the child). In actuality, everyone within the family is suffering the pain of the diagnosis of the hearing loss and attention needs to be paid to the entire system. In order for the child to be successful, he or she needs to be within a family that is nurturing and functioning as optimally as possible.

There are characteristics of the optimum family discussed within the therapy literature that are useful in understanding what makes a family system function well. These are idealized family characteristics. No family will be able to incorporate all of these to perfection. Satir's book (1971), *People Making,* describes many of the characteristics of the ideal family and Napier and Whitaker's book (1978), The Family Crucible, details the way therapists work with the family unit. While both books are old, they are classics and may be read with profit by the interested reader. The website for the American Association of Marriage and Family Therapists (*www.aamft.org*) provides contemporary information on therapeutic approaches to families in stress.

Clear Communication

Almost any therapist who writes about family systems is concerned with the patterns of communication within the family. Dysfunctional families have implied communication in which much is "understood" but not said. These are silent "rules" that a family follows that are usually understood by every one in the system. For example, a family may decide not to talk about how they feel regarding their child's hearing loss. If there's an implicit directive that emotions are unacceptable, family members often feel isolated in their pain. A child's hearing loss causes high expressing emotions to flourish within the family, not only for the parents, but for siblings and grandparents as well. If the family has no mechanism for talking about their feelings, the family system is stressed. This can take many forms. For example, the unexpressed and unacknowledged anger is often displaced on another family member. The angry person does not recognize the source of the anger as the repressed feelings about the hearing loss. Conflicts in dysfunctional families are seldom about what they're really angry over because parents lack the skills for direct non-threatening confrontation.

Another common emotion in less than optimal families is guilt. If not acknowledged, it leads to super dedication and overprotection of the child. This leaves little time for siblings or energy to maintain the marriage. A healthy family system would allow for clear direct communication where both feeling and content are expressed.

Overlapping Roles

In order for a family system to function well, each member needs to assume a role. In an optimally functioning family, roles are delegated based on ability and interest. In less than optimal families, roles are assigned on beliefs such as gender or age regardless of competency. In a given family, for example, the wife may be the better earner and the husband the better cook, but because of their values roles are assigned based on gender. So he's the wage earner and she's the cook. This may not be optimal for this family.

The optimal family also has the fail-safe mechanism of overlapping roles so that if one family member is absent or ailing other members can fill in. This enables the family to function when under stress, such as when a spouse becomes disabled or a child has a hearing loss. When there is stress on a family, roles need to be reshuffled in order for the family to function. Parental energy, at least in the early stages of diagnosis of hearing loss, is redirected to the child with the hearing loss. Someone within the family system needs to fill in those other functions that the parents no longer have the energy to perform. The grandparents, an aunt, or older siblings, usually come to the fore. If they cannot, the family system is at risk. Ultimately, there's a long-term reshuffling of roles as well. Usually the mother takes on the major responsibility for the education of the child and this leaves a vacuum in fulfilling some of her other responsibilities.

With overlapping roles, an optimum fully intact family can adjust relatively easily to the stress of hearing loss in the child. If the mother, for example, normally has the role of shopping and preparing dinner, she may not be able to do this while assuming the task of managing her child's greater needs due to the hearing loss. In an optimal family system, others can fill in this role leaving the mother free to devote additional energy to the child. If the mother tries to assume additional responsibilities of managing the child's hearing loss without shedding any of her other responsibilities, her stress level can adversely affect how the family functions.

Intimacy

In an optimal family, the members feel loved and valued. Home is where we should feel supported, loved, and above all else emotionally safe. Families have different ways of expressing love. Some express it physically while others are more subtle. The caring within the family needs to be communicated in a way that the members can perceive it. An optimal family provides intimacy while respecting the need for space. It's cohesive without being enmeshed. In less than optimal families, members may feel unloved or neglected. This is especially true of siblings of special needs children. So much family energy is directed to the child with the hearing loss that the other children often feel unloved, neglected and unimportant.

Conflict Mediation

The process of raising children is inherently conflicted. The parent's responsibility is to set boundaries for the child. The child's biological mandate is to push against the boundaries imposed by the parents. In families with a special needs child, guilt often blurs these boundaries creating an enmeshed family system. The parents try to compensate for the child's handicap by giving in where they wouldn't with siblings. It becomes difficult to distinguish between normal development issues like childhood manipulation and those really attributable to the handicap. Parents can have a tendency to waver on the boundaries or help the child so much that the child doesn't learn self-responsibility. Eventually, this can create a child who doesn't feel secure because the rules are not clear. The child doesn't know how to operate in the world and take responsibility for his or her actions. This child can easily grow up to be like the man in Chapter 1 who wouldn't move so he could see the signer, but instead chose to blame the lecturer.

It's the job of the parents to teach conflict resolution and responsibility, modeling it themselves and gradually rewarding self-responsibility with more freedom until the child achieves adulthood. In a healthy family system, conflict is dealt with through people listening to one another and coming to solutions together that are fair and safe for the child. In less than optimal families, conflict is discouraged because it's seen as a threat to the family system. The person who has the power usually resolves the conflicts by the threat of force. Children are expected to listen to parents solely because they are the parents, and because of their dependency, children are vulnerable to physical threats or to the withdrawal of support. The suppression of the conflict usually leads to passive-aggressive behavior. Children learn not to confront authority directly but rather to subvert it by passive means. It is then not a question of whether conflict is present in a family, but always a matter of how the family deals with conflict.

Managing Change

Families are like any entity; subject to constantly changing forces. A family system is similar to a man walking across a tightrope. In order to get across he must constantly make small adjustments. So too with the family, adjustments must be made to a constantly changing reality. Children grow and require greater freedom, parents age and require more help. Then there are the external factors that can beset families, such as loss of job, change in location, illness, and so forth. A child's hearing loss is one of those external forces mandating change within the family. If the other optimal factors are present, such as clear and direct communication, role flexibility, intimacy, and conflict resolution skills, then the change becomes much easier for the family to manage than if they were absent. Change is never easy. It involves an adaptation from everyone within the family system. This is the teaching aspect of hearing loss. We bring to life what life demands of us and a child's hearing loss demands new roles and new skills. In the adaptation there is learning. The same is true for the family system. If it can accommodate to the change mandated by the child with hearing loss, then the family will grow with new skills and knowledge acquired by everyone. If it cannot change, then the family may dissolve or wallow in dysfunction.

Marital Pair

Marriage is usually the lynchpin around which the family functions. It is where partners should receive nurturing and support in order to cope with the demands of child rearing. Single parents can and do successfully raise their children. They usually do this within a supportive context of other family friends or hired help.

Where there's a child with hearing loss, the demands on parenting are more severe. Professionals within programs will need to be especially supportive in single-family homes. I've seen divorced families be successful, such as in joint custody agreements where both parents share commitment to the child. This is relatively rare since most of the time one parent is left with the responsibility of managing the child's hearing loss. As I look back on what makes a child with a hearing loss successful, an important variable (there are many) is the strength and consistency of the support they receive from parents—married or not.

Marriages in successful two-parent families are

usually complimentary. We tend to seek in our marital partner that which is missing in ourselves. Sometimes we do this consciously, but more often it's done unconsciously. For example, a marital partner who is emotional may seek someone who is more cognitively oriented. This gives a completeness or congruence to the couple that neither partner may have.

In a successful long-term relationship, the partners rub off on one another, there is a mutual learning, and each becomes more congruent. In the short term when the couple is under stress, the differences in coping can grate. Couples will almost always grieve at different rates. If one is emotionally upset, the other can feel it is necessary to hold it together by being "strong." In this scenario, the partner who is upset often does not appreciate the complimentary nature of the role the spouse is playing and is dismayed that the partner is not equally upset.

Grieving

In one family that I worked with in a support group, the wife was especially upset and she grieved for a long time. She grew up in a large family and her immediate older sister had a severe hearing loss. Since this sister got most of the little family attention that was available, she was often jealous and not very nice to her sister. Her mother often said to her, "If you're not nice to your sister, God will punish you." Now that she had a child with hearing loss she *knew* that God was punishing her and hence she bore deep feelings of grief and guilt. As she gained some perspective on her emotional reaction, she tried to share her feelings with her husband within the group. However, he seemed incapable of grasping the reality of their child's hearing loss. Any assurances he offered that their daughter would be okay felt meaningless to her.

She came to the support group one day and reported, "A funny thing happened last night. I was making supper and I had the radio on while I was cooking. My husband came home and told me to turn down the radio because I would wake the baby. I told him you could not wake the baby. She can't hear. He got a funny expression on his face and then he started to cry. He cried all night. I've never seen him like that."

My comment to her was, "It seems that you've been feeling pretty good lately, and now it's his turn to feel badly." In this case, the husband had to be relieved of his protector role before he could begin to access his pain. This often requires a great deal of counseling as many men carry the cultural burden of being the strong, silent protector.

Shared Values

The successful marriage is one in which there are shared values. Couples need to be on the same page as to the big picture. When there are basic agreements about their values then decisions, as a couple are relatively easy to make. Shared values are an important unifying factor. They enable the couple to prioritize and recognize what is important, especially when it comes to raising the children.

Parents of children with normal hearing seldom have to think about most educational decisions they make. They have their own educational experience to draw upon. The parents of children with hearing loss are in uncharted territory and constantly confronted with decisions in areas where they have no experience. One of the first decisions, for example, will be on the choice of an early intervention program and communication methodology. Another choice is whether to have a cochlear implant for their child. These decisions are occurring now at a very early stage in the parenting process often with first time parents. These decisions bring to the fore parental values and if there is little agreement between the parents then there will be added stress on their relationship as they try to work out their differences.

Decisions regarding the child with a hearing loss have a profound effect on everyone in the family. For example, the decision to relocate is frequently made based on the child's schooling, which may not always benefit other members of the family. This is when clear communication is needed to try to find a solution that has some benefit for everyone in the family.

Marital Stress

Ironically, clinical programs frequently increase marital stress. So much of parental education is in reality "mother" education. The mother then is often so far ahead of her husband in what she knows about hearing loss and in child management that she becomes dismayed at his incompetence. This usually does not go over too well with the husband and conflict can ensue.

Hearing loss in a child can often add stress to the marital pair. From that stress growth can take place and couples can become stronger. It can lead to recognition of their individual strengths. One husband commented, "I never knew she had this kind of strength. She has taken on the education system and won." The wife found that he really cared about her and their son. He went to the meetings and was her support.

The Siblings

One of the first topics that emerges in parent support groups is concern for the siblings with normal hearing. Parents are often very aware that siblings are given little time or attention around the time of diagnosis—a feeling shared by many siblings. Research indicates that having a child with a disability in the family has a mixed effect on the siblings (Grossman, 1972; Darius, 1988). There are positives as well as negatives. Much depends on how well parents are able to adjust to the reality of the hearing loss in their child. The child most affected is usually the oldest girl and the least affected is the oldest boy. Parental expectations for female children are so very different than for male children. Often the oldest female child is burdened with care-giving responsibility that an oldest son might not have.

Below are excerpts from a letter written to me by the oldest female sibling of a brother with a severe hearing loss:

Dear Dr Luterman:

I have a lot of feelings about Robert's loss of hearing and how it has affected me. I've told my mother only some of my feelings because she gets upset or angry when I say how I felt when I was little. I don't know if it's because she thinks that I'm saying she wasn't a good mother to me or why she gets upset.

I think when I was little I had very mixed feelings. I felt very jealous of Robert. I can remember feeling very neglected because I always thought that he got all the attention from everybody. Of course now I realize my mother had to work with him more and it was all necessary, but I didn't understand that when I was little. I remember wishing that I was deaf for awhile thinking then I'd have to go into the hospital and everyone would bring me presents and give me more attention. I even remember trying to break my arm by jumping out of my treehouse (which never happened). I've never told my mother any of this.

I also remember being very proud of Robert, attending his school plays and having tears come to my eyes when I watched him on stage. I remember wanting to be friends with his friends. I also remember people saying mean things about people with hearing loss in general, like they can't talk and feeling so hurt and intimidated that I couldn't even stand up for him. I usually just said nothing.

I think Robert's hearing loss created a lot of extra tension in my parents' marriage. I remember my mother getting really upset about the taxis taking him to school, some school problem, and other things. I remember my father not wanting or just not getting involved and my mother getting upset at him. I really never understood just how it affected my father but I know it was real hard on my mother.

I guess the way I dealt with my jealousy was by deciding to work with deaf children when I grew up. I decided this ever since I used to go watch Robert at Emerson College through the one-way mirror with my mother. And here I am, a speech pathologist working at a school where the total communication class is housed, and I love working with the kids, ages 5-12.
Sincerely,
Sara

Grossman (1972) and Darius (1988) address "negatives" and "positives" that normal hearing siblings experience. I want to present some of them to help you better understand possible family dynamics that could be occurring with your own children.

1. Feeling Neglected

This issue generally relates to lack of attention in the family as noted by Sara. There's a limited amount of energy in a family system and when a disproportionate amount goes to the child with a hearing loss, normal hearing siblings often feel the lack of attention. Therefore, Sara considers falling out of a tree to break her arm so she can get some attention. She also found it hard to talk to her mother about her feelings. This happens frequently in families with a child with a hearing loss because many parents are in denial about the sibling's negative emotions. Conversely, other parents may feel guilty because of the lack of attention they're able to give to the other children.

2. Feeling Family has Enough Problems—
They had to be Perfect

Many siblings feel that they have to be especially good and conforming because parents are so stressed coping with the needs of the child with a hearing loss. Sara noticed the stress on her parents and knew they couldn't handle a whole lot more.

3. Felt They Lost their Youth due to Added
Responsibilities

As the oldest girl Sara was also burdened with responsibilities early in life by either caring for her brother or babysitting the other siblings. Many siblings with normal hearing feel that as a consequence of assuming responsibility so early in their lives they lost their youth.

4. Shame about a Special Needs Child and the Guilt

The normal hearing sibling often has a sense of embarrassment. One sibling for example, hated to go into McDonalds because everyone looked at them because his brother wore hearing aids. The family needs to support the idea that there is no shame to it.

5. Concern that it might Happen to Them

The hearing loss is also a source of anxiety to children with normal hearing as they often worry about losing their own hearing. One oldest female sibling, for example, wondered if she would have a child with hearing loss. She also assumed she would have to be the caretaker for her brother after her parents died.

6. Survivor Guilt

Siblings frequently have "survivor guilt" by wondering why they have normal hearing and their sibling does not. This is not unusual or unexpected.

Grossman and Darius also reported positive experiences:

1. Increased Sense of Self-Worth

Positives for siblings included feeling important and needed because the parents incorporated them into activities that helped the child with a hearing loss to learn language or listening skills. Many siblings, in fact, became the prime home therapist and many became the home and school interpreter. Several siblings tutored their brother or sister in school all of which contributed to an increased sense of self-worth.

2. Greater Understanding and Compassion for People with Disabilities

They felt able to understand prejudice better and many felt that the family became closer and stronger in their common bond to cope with the hearing impairment. Most siblings developed a respect for minorities and the underdog because in most cases they were a minority and an underdog. This helped them to be accepting of differences in others.

3. Vocational Direction

Many, as did Sara, have found a new vocational direction. Often speech therapists, teachers of the deaf, audiologists and interpreters are themselves siblings of children with hearing impairments. The skills they learned as siblings were very valuable in training programs for a professional working with the hearing impaired, they were often ahead of many of their classmates.

4. Increased Appreciation of their own Good Health

Many siblings felt blessed and fortunate that they had escaped a disability. We seldom appreciate our good health until we lose it. Siblings of children with hearing loss seldom go a day without appreciating their capacity to hear.

The Grandparents

The influence of grandparents is in every family whether they are present or not. We always carry our family of origin into our new nuclear family. Our ideas about being a parent and being a spouse are forged in our family of origin by watching and experiencing our parents. We often vow not to be like them and then find often to our dismay that we say and do many of the same things they did.

Grandparenthood can be a marvelous state. It is a time when the grandparent can experience all the joys of parenting without any of the responsibilities. The grandparent can provide unconditional regard for the child. Parenting I think is a job that no one does entirely to his or her own satisfaction. I think you can get there with the grandparenting.

Despite their sometimes physical remoteness, grandparents are usually severely impacted by the child's hearing loss. For them it is a double loss. They are hurting for their child and for their grandchild. They are often in denial much longer than the parents are (Lowe, 1989) since it's easier to stay in denial when one doesn't have the day-to-day responsibilities of child management. This situation often creates a role reversal crisis between the parent and grandparent. Even in adulthood many of us turn to our parents for support and help in times of crisis.

When the parent turns to the grandparent for the support they crave, at the time of diagnosis it is usually not there. The parent has so much more information and is further down the road to acceptance than the grandparent that a role reversal often takes place. The parents, instead of receiving support, often have to give it. This very often leaves the parent feeling disappointed and angry. A predictable life crisis occurs when we have to start parenting our parents. Normally this crisis is fueled by years of little incidents where we recognize our parents' increasing incompetence. When there's a child with hearing loss in the family, the crisis comes on quite suddenly and much sooner than either parent or grandparent is prepared for. This leaves grandparents bewildered and parents feeling very much alone.

Many times there's not good communication of feelings between grandparents and parents and many unresolved issues from the past come to the fore. Several different scenarios are often played out. The grandparents, for example, express their concern by asking if the parent had considered a possible avenue of therapy or cure which the parent hears as a question of their competency. From the grandparents point of view it's a simple question. For the parent it's a reminder of their childhood experience of having their competency questioned.

In another case, grandparents are afraid to say anything about how they're feeling because they don't want to burden their child with their own emotional pain. The parent, on the other hand, assumes the grandparent is indifferent and is upset and angry that their parent is not concerned and not emotionally supportive. Again, implicit communication creates so many difficulties in relationships.

Parents often feel that they have disappointed their parents by giving birth to a child with hearing loss. One of the implicit contracts that parents have with their children is to produce grandchildren that will bring pleasure and joy to them. A child with special needs brings pain (there is joy but it's hard to find especially in the early stages of acceptance). And parents frequently feel that they've failed their own parents. Anger often masks the guilt that the parent feels and an unhealthy dynamic begins to develop in the parent/grandparent relationship. The anger based on guilt can take many forms as it is often displaced. Parents are angry because the grandparent cannot seem to manage the hearing aids thus limiting the babysitting that they ordinarily might provide. Grandparents, on the other hand, often acutely feel they're failing their child and are confused about how to help. One grandmother commented, "I always feel like I'm walking on eggshells with my daughter. She might explode at me at anytime."

I've yet to find a grandparent who didn't want to help or for that matter, a family that did not need help. The solution often is in helping the family communicate their needs better within an emotionally safe environment. This is something professionals need to provide. To be sure, there are families where there is minimal conflict between parents and grandparents and the grandparents are an enormous support and asset. Usually these families are well functioning to begin with and have a high degree of communication and intimacy.

The hearing loss can also be a very positive factor in the parent/grandparent relationship. I remember one grandmother commenting that she had come to admire her daughter by seeing her strength in coping with the hearing loss. Prior to that time, she had thought her daughter was shallow. Here again there's a differential effect of the impact that hearing loss can have on a family. It can work to be a unifying and positive experience for everyone or it can push a marginal family into dysfunction.

Grandparents can be role models as many grandparents wear hearing aids and thus the grandchild can identify with the grandparent. Both can learn to wear their hearing aids with pride. I remember one family where the grandfather was reluctant to wear his aids until he was enlisted as a role model for his grand-son.

Grandparents can also provide parents with respite care and they can be surrogate parents to the hearing siblings. Professionals need to pay attention to the grandparents. It is energy well spent. Grandparents are usually the most emotionally isolated family members. They seldom get an opportunity to meet and talk to other grandparents. Within the Emerson program (Luterman, 1999) we make every effort to reach out to grandparents by providing a grandparent support group.

The Successful Family

Several research studies have been conducted to determine which factors will lead to a successful outcome for a child with a disability (Lavell and Keogh, 1980; Venters, 1981; Gallagher et. al., 1981). None of these studies looked specifically at families with hearing loss. The issue of adaptation to a disability ("success") is not disability specific. The design of the studies was the same regardless of disability. Professionals working with the families were asked to rate them as to successful or not. Where there was unanimity of agreement among the professionals, researchers interviewed the families in depth. Successful families appeared to have some characteristics in common. They felt empowered in that they could make a difference in the child's life. In particular, the mother felt empowered. These mothers became strong advocates for their children, found the most suitable program for their child and utilized the skills of the professionals involved.

These findings are similar to the results of Schlessinger's (1994) study cited earlier who found that mothers with high self-esteem were most successful in facilitating their child's literacy development.

A family must make philosophical sense of hearing loss. They must be able to answer the question to their satisfaction—Why us? If they cannot find a satisfactory answer, they become mired in bitterness and resentment. This question often leads to discussion about the influence of a greater power (i.e., God) and a re-evaluation of the family's cosmology. Answers are individual for each family. In a support group discussion, one mother said, "Since this happened I've been to church every day." Sitting across from her, another said, "Since this happened I've been so angry with God I've not been able to go to church." Each family needs to find an explanation as to why bad things can happen to good people (Kushner, 1983).

The traditional Judeo-Christian view held by many in our society is that God is in heaven punishing the wicked and rewarding the good. Therefore, if I have a child with a hearing loss I must have been wicked or God is wicked. Neither position is very tenable. Families must find some way to reach peace of mind and heart for there are many roads, all of them unique and individual.

The key to a successful integration of hearing loss into a family is the degree to which parents are able to integrate hearing loss into their lives. If hearing loss is seen as a tragedy and a terrible loss, the family system will be continually assaulted by the negative emotions and siblings will be at risk. If it's treated as a teacher for everyone, and the positive aspects of hearing loss are seen and noted, then siblings can flourish. The ability to see positives in what might be an otherwise dire situation is known as reframing. It is a skill we all need to develop in order to live a healthy and happy life.

References

Darius, B. (1988). A Study of the Siblings of Hearing Impaired Children - How they were Affected by the Handicap. Boston: Emerson College, Unpublished Masters Thesis.

Gallagher, J., Cross, A. and Sharfman,W. (1981). Parental adaptation to a handicapped child: The father's role. Journal of Division of Early Childhood 3, 3-14.

Grossman, E.K. (1972). *Brothers and Sisters of Retarded Children.* Syracuse, NY: University Press.

Kushner, H.S. (1983). *When Bad Things Happen to Good People.* New York, NY: Avon Books.

Lavall, K. and Keogh, B. (1980). Expectation and attribution of parents of handicapped children. In: *Parents and Families of Handicapped Children.* J. J. Gallagher (Ed.), San Francisco: Jossey- Bass.

Lowe, T. (1989). *Grandparents View the Hearing Impaired Child.* Boston, MA: Emerson College, Unpublished Master's Thesis.

Luterman, D. (1999). *The Young Deaf Child.* Baltimore, MD: York Press.

Minuchin, S. (1974). *Families and Family Therapy.* Cambridge, MA: Harvard University Press.

Napier, A and Whitaker, C. (1978). *The Family Crucible.* New York, NY: Harper and Row.

Satir, V. (1971). *People Making.* Palo Alto, CA: Science and Behavior Books.

Schlessinger, H. (1994). The Elusive X Factor: Parental Contributions to Literacy. In: *A Free Hand,* M. Walworth, D. Moores, T. O'Rourke (Eds.). Silver Springs, MD: TJ Publishers.

Venters, M. (1981). Families Coping with Chronic and Severe Childhood Illness. The Case of Cystic Fibrosis. Social Science and Medicine 15A, 289-97.

Chapter 3

Hearing Aids and Cochlear Implants

Linda Thibodeau, Ph. D.

Dr. Linda Thibodeau is a Professor at the University of Texas at Dallas since 1996 where she co-directs the Pediatric Aural Habilitation Training Specialist Project. Prior to that she worked at The University of Texas at Austin, at the University of Texas Speech and Hearing Institute, in otolaryngology clinics and in the public schools. She teaches in the areas of Amplification and Pediatric Aural Habilitation. Her research at the Advanced Hearing Research Center of the Callier Center for Communication Disorders involves evaluation of the speech perception of listeners with hearing loss and auditory processing problems as well as evaluation of amplification systems and hearing assistance technology to help those persons.

She consults with several school districts and manufacturers regarding FM arrangements in the classroom. Her professional interests include serving as the co-chair of the the ANSI committee to develop a standard for the Electroacoustic Evaluation of ALDs; and serving as Editor-in-Chief of the Journal of the Academy of Rehabilitative Audiology, and Associate Editor for the American Journal of Audiology.

Perhaps the most challenging decision that a parent must make for their child with a hearing loss is how they will communicate. Most parents choose a communication method that relies on auditory input provided through some type of amplification or alternate stimulation, such as a cochlear implant. Research has shown that neuronal connections are rapidly forming during the first years of life, so that the sooner the amplification or cochlear implants are provided, the more likely the child will develop normally functioning acoustic pathways (Sininger, Doyle, & Moore,1999). Typically hearing aids will be the first consideration regardless of the child's age. Bringing sound to the child either through amplification or a cochlear implant will be equally important whether the family is using only speech to communicate or a combination of speech and sign language.

If the child is receiving limited benefit from hearing aids after a four-to-six month trial and the child is over 12 months of age, a cochlear implant may be considered. One situation in which cochlear implants would be recommended without a hearing aid trial would be when a child has suffered a hearing loss as a result of meningitis (an infection of the tissue linings of the brain and/or spinal cord). Because bony growth in the inner ear may occur after meningitis and could affect the proper insertion of the implant, a cochlear implant may be recommended within a few months of the child's recovery. During the course of the journey parents will meet many professionals. Among them are:

1) Otologists or otolaryngologists: Medical doctors who treat ear, nose, and/or throat problems and perform cochlear implant surgeries;

2) Audiologists: Professionals who fit and/or provide hearing aids, cochlear implants, and hearing assistive technology that aid reception of sound;

3) Speech-Language Pathologists: Therapists who teach the child and family how to develop communication consistent with developmental expectations;

4) Educators: Parent-infant advisors who come into the home or teachers in the classroom who facilitate early communication, cognitive, social, and physical development; and

5) Parents: Others who have already been through many of the challenges can often respond to the concerns and celebrations in a context of their own experiences.

Some or all of these professionals will be involved in the selection and use of the hearing aids or cochlear implants. Therefore, one may consider this the beginning of a new journey with new techniques of travel and caring hosts to meet along the way. As with any journey, there are many decisions to make and much information to gather ahead of time or along the way that will hopefully lead to not only quick but comfortable travel. The process begins with the audiological diagnosis followed by the selection of each type of device. In addition to hearing aids and cochlear implants, hearing assistive technology will often be needed to help compensate for reduced sound when there is distance from the speaker or interfering background noise.

Success with amplification, cochlear implants or assistive technology will depend on not only the expertise of hearing care providers to match the features of the technology to the needs of the child, but also the psychological acceptance of the devices by the family. The introduction of technology with a positive regard for the benefits it can provide is critical. Depending on the age of the child and his or her siblings, there may be opportunities to explain how hearing aids are needed by some, like glasses or braces are needed by others. When children develop a focus that the hearing devices are tools to access information rather than a mark of abnormality, they will be establishing a means to address challenging communication situations with openness and assertiveness. Because even the most sophisticated hearing aids or cochlear implants do not restore perfect hearing, children will need positive coping skills in addition to the technology to maximize communication.

Hearing Aids

Whether a child uses a hearing aid or a cochlear implant, it is important to understand that these devices are aids to access acoustic information. In some respects, hearing aids function much like radios. Typically, all radios have two controls with very distinct functions, one to control the volume and one to tune in the station. These controls can be thought of as representing the two major effects of hearing loss, a reduction in loudness and a reduction in clarity. The loudness effect can be simulated by a reduction in the volume control and the clarity effect can be simulated by slightly mistuning the station so there is "fuzziness" to the signal. Hearing aids can easily restore the loudness of the signal. However, restoring clarity may be more difficult. Just as the controls on a radio can be adjusted independently, you may have two similar degrees of hearing loss but very different perceptions of clarity. It is possible that even though loudness has been restored, the hearing aid may not be capable of restoring clarity. This is certainly an oversimplification of the audiological issues addressed by hearing aids. Amplification options can be very complex and optimal performance requires expertise in at least five areas: audiological evaluation, selecting the device, hearing aid fitting, evaluation of hearing aid benefit, and counseling the family on use and operation.

The decision to obtain hearing aids is determined by the audiologist and parents at the time of diagnosis. Even children with mild losses are candidates for amplification because of the critical need to hear the sounds of speech for language development. Many language concepts, for example, depend on hearing one of the softest speech sounds, the "s." When this sound is not heard, a child may have difficulty with plurals, possessives, and present tense verbs. For school-aged children, hearing all sounds of speech with a mild loss is difficult because the typical classroom noise may mask, or cover up, the soft speech sounds.

Audiologists

Being fitted with hearing aids requires the expertise of a licensed audiologist or hearing instrument specialist (HIS). Those who hold a Certificate of Clinical Competence (CCC) have obtained a Master's Degree and passed a national examination. As of this time (2006) the profession of Audiology is transitioning and the professional Docotor of Audiology (Au.D.) will replace the Master's Degree as the "entry level" degree. Virtually all states have licensure or registration requirements and hearing care providers must maintain their license by obtaining annual continuing education credits. Audiologists may have their own private practice or work in a hospital, physician's office, government health facility, university or school. Hearing aids may also be obtained from Hearing Instrument Specialists who are individuals who have met state licensure requirements which typically include completing high school, passing a state examination and having practical experience with a licensed provider.

In order to find an audiologist, one may consult a phone directory or state licensure board to look for those with the professional credentials. Organizations that can search for a certified audiologist in your area include the American Academy of Audiology (*www.audiology.org:* 1-800-AAA-2336), the Academy of Dispensing Audiologists (*www.audiol ogy.org:* 1-866-493-5544). or the American Speech, Language, and Hearing Association (*www.asha.org:* 1-800-638-8255).

Choosing a hearing care provider is a very important initial step in obtaining hearing aids. Issues to consider are if they provide hearing assistive technology to interface with the hearing aids, and whether adequate loaner equipment would be provided when personal equipment must be repaired. Audiological facilities may also be selected based on insurance reimbursement programs, payment options, and scheduling flexibility. It will also be important to work with an audiologist who will provide regular updates to medical and educational personnel. For example, by sending copies of diagnostic reports to the child's doctor, teacher or speech pathologist, the intervention can be coordinated among them. The child with a hearing loss will be optimally served when the professionals can function as a team with a common goal to maximize auditory information for communication development.

Audiological Evaluation

The process of obtaining a hearing aid starts with the audiological evaluation. Through a variety of techniques, the hearing ability of children can be evaluated regardless of age. Some techniques require no response from the child, such as auditory brainstem response where the responses to sound are determined through the use of electrodes placed on the scalp while the child sleeps or sits very quietly. Others involve a small probe placed in the ear to measure responses to sound to evaluate functioning of the middle ear through a test called *tympanometry*, or functioning of the inner ear through a test called *otoacoustic emissions.* Prior to any of these procedures, an examination of the outer ear should be made using an otoscope to determine any wax obstructions or auditory canal abnormalities that would affect the hearing aid fitting.

Behavioral responses to sound can also be determined in a soundbooth with specific stimuli and games to encourage the child to respond by looking at toy lights near the speaker or dropping toys in a bucket. Infants and young children are often seated on a parent's lap and older children typically sit at a small table. Ideally, the child can wear headphones or ear inserts to deliver the sound so that ear-specific information can be obtained. When children don't tolerate the headphones, the stimuli are delivered through soundfield loudspeakers. Responses represent the hearing ability of the "better" ear.

Throughout all these tests, the audiologist is trying to determine the softest level of sound that causes a response across a range of pitches from very low to very high pitch sounds. This softest response level is called threshold and is quantified in *Decibels* (dB) which are units of sound. A comparison is also made between responses to sounds presented through the air conduction pathway (earphones), and those presented through the bone conduction pathway (a bone vibrator placed behind the ear). By comparing these responses, the audiologist can help determine if the hearing loss is the result of some problem in the outer or middle ear, which can often be treated by an oto-laryngologist, or in the inner ear or central auditory pathways, which is generally not reversible.

These responses to sound are plotted on a graph called the *audiogram* that will guide the audiologist in recommending amplification. As shown on the audiogram in Figure 3-1, the level of sounds is represented as decibels hearing level (dB HL) down the side and the pitch is represented as frequency (Hz) across the top. The quietest sounds one can hear are represented near the top of the audiogram and the loudest sounds at the bottom. Note, "0 dB hearing level" is not an absence of sound, rather it represents the level that persons with normal hearing can hear about half the time. Some persons with exceptionally good hearing can respond to tones at -5 or even -10 dB HL. Low-pitched sounds are on the left side of the audiogram (e.g. 250 Hz) and high-pitched sounds are on the right side (e.g. 8000 Hz). The thresholds from the earphones for the right and left ears are plotted as "o" and "x," respectively; whereas "<" and ">" represent thresholds from the bone vibrator.

The speech signal is composed of pitches in the mid range (e.g. 500, 1000, and 2000 Hz). The thresholds at these frequencies are averaged to provide what is called the pure-tone average (PTA). When

Figure 3-1: Audiogram of a child with a severe sensorineural hearing loss bilaterally. The circles and x's represent responses for the right and left ears, respectively. The open arrows represent responses to bone conduction for the left.

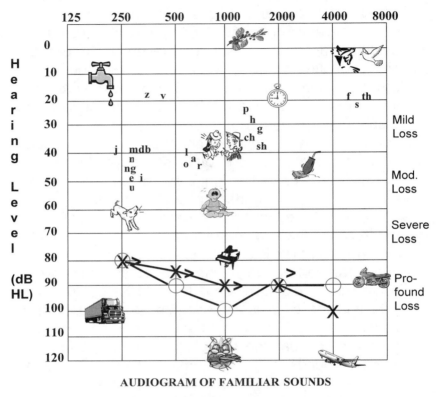

AUDIOGRAM OF FAMILIAR SOUNDS

FREQUENCY IN CYCLES PER SECOND (Hz)

responses are obtained at levels 20 dB HL or less, hearing is considered normal. Degrees of hearing loss are shown on the right in Figure 3-1. For example, if the PTA is between 20 and 40 dB HL, the hearing loss is considered to be mild, while a PTA between 71 and 90 dB HL is considered to be severe. The approximate levels and pitches for speech and other sounds are also shown on the audiogram. Because the mid-frequency speech sounds have more intensity than the high-frequency sounds, the general shape of the area represented by the sounds of speech is known as the speech banana. The audiogram of a child with a severe sensorineural loss in the right and left ears is plotted in Figure 3-1.

This child did not respond to sound until it reached levels of 80 to 100 dB HL. By looking at these thresholds in relation to the speech sounds in Figure 3-1 (the speech banana), it can be determined that none of these speech sounds would be audible to this child without a hearing aid.

[Examples of hearing loss simulations for different audiograms are provided in Information for Parents of Children with Hearing Loss available at: *http://www.ut dallas.edu/~thib/rehabinfo*. A unique hearing loss simulator to explore the effects of different degrees of hearing loss is available at the National Institute for Occupational Safety and Health website: *http://holme ssafety.org/hlsim*]

Selecting the Device

The audiogram is the basis for selection of many aspects of the hearing aid. In addition to the power of the aid, there are several operational features that must be considered for each individual situation. Regardless of these features, the basic operation including main parts, batteries and coupling is similar for all aids. Furthermore, in selecting amplification, it is important to remember that two aids should always be considered unless there are audiological or physical reasons to fit only one ear. This binaural fitting is the optimal arrangement for children in order to gain access to as much auditory information as possible while developing speech and language.

Basic Operation of Hearing Aids

All hearing aids have four main components: a microphone, amplifier, receiver and power supply. The microphone converts the acoustic air waves into an electrical signal. The electrical signal is then changed in the amplifier to give more emphasis in the high or low pitches depending on the child's loss, but the basic form of the signal resembles that of the acoustic energy in the input signal. This emphasis is known as *gain* of the aid. Gain can be thought of as an increase in the level of the output of the hearing aid relative to the level of the input. The final stage is the receiver where the electrical output from the amplifier is converted back to audible sound and delivered into the ear canal. The hearing aid requires small batteries to operate that usually last about 10 days.

As shown in Figure 3-2, the optimal style of hearing aids for young children consists of two parts, the earmold and the behind-the-ear (BTE) aid. There are smaller, one-component hearing aids such as in-the-ear or in-the-canal aids. These are not recommended for children younger than 15 years old because they would need to be remade frequently as the child's ears grow and they do not allow room for features such as FM receivers that are very important for a child to hear in noisy environments. Other features that cannot be included in smaller custom-made hearing aids are T-coils, accessible switches and controls, direct auditory input and/or longer lasting batteries.

Considerable research has been conducted to determine the optimal amount of amplification needed across the frequency range to hear all the cues of speech (Seewald, Moodie, & Sinclair, 1999). Computer programs are used to calculate the desired gain based on the child's thresholds, age, and ear canal size. This stage is the most critical part of the hearing aid evaluation because it requires precise adjustments and verification to ensure the power is sufficient for the child but not too extreme so that the sound is uncomfortable. The acoustic signal can also be optimized for the child through modifications to the earmold such as a widened opening or a short canal to provide additional emphasis to the high pitches.

Figure 3-2: Behind-the-ear hearing aid with earmold attached.

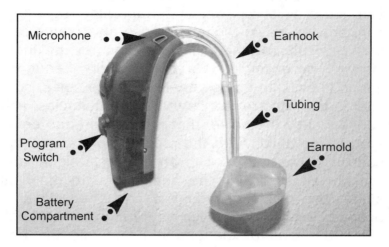

[There are many features offered on hearing aids by a variety of manufacturers. Many manufacturers of hearing aids can be located through www.audiologyonline.com]

Hearing Aid Options

Advancements in hearing aids are being made rapidly and many of the common problems of traditional aids from the 1970s and 1980s have been solved. With digital technology becoming more common, there are many more options for parents to consider. For example, the high-pitched squealing sound known as feedback that could occur with powerful hearing aids can now often be reduced or eliminated through digital processing. In addition, directionality of the microphones and noise reduction programs are also options which can improve the quality of the signal.

Digital Signal Processing (DSP) hearing aids currently represent nearly 90% of all new hearing aid sales in 2006. Similar to an analog aid, the acoustic signal is converted into an electric signal via a microphone in a DSP aid. Then the electric signal is converted into a code of zeros and ones that can represent the changes in acoustic energy in the input signal. This code of numbers can be manipulated to provide more or less power in certain pitch regions in very precise ways. Digital aids can also create certain processing schemes depending on the input signal. For example, if a constant low-frequency sound is analyzed, it is very likely to be noise, so a filter is activated to reduce the low frequencies, and consequently the noise, that is amplified and delivered to the child. After the processing is done, the code is converted back to an electrical signal and transduced similar to the analog aid. In the final stage, the electrical signal is converted back to acoustic energy and delivered through the earhook into the tubing of the earmold and into the ear. Digital technology allows for many settings that must be determined for each child and is now priced comparable to analog hearing aids depending on the features selected.

There are at least nine important considerations that parents should know about when selecting amplification which include:

1) multiple programs
2) directional microphones
3) compression
4) noise reduction circuitry
5) FM compatibility
6) T-coil reception
7) child appropriate features
8) one versus two hearing aids
9) feedback reduction

With the rapid changes in technology, there will always be new features to consider, but the nine presented here will likely continue to be considerations.

1) *Multiple Programs*

As with most technology, there is a range of sophistication in hearing aids and one of the most flexible features to consider is multiple programs. Having this feature allows you to basically have two or three hearing aids within one case. In addition to having different amounts of gain in each program, there may be different types of noise reduction, and different features such as FM reception or T-coil. Typically, the programs have different amplification characteristics for different listening environments, such as conversations in quiet or riding in a car. When the aid is turned on, it always begins in the default program. As the toggle switch is moved, the user will typically hear beeps to signal the change to a new program. Parents may find that using a remote control to change programs in both aids simultaneously is much easier than chasing a toddler to find a switch on each aid. Program 1 may be comfortable listening in quiet such as at home reading a book, while Program 2 may allow noise reduction for listening in the classroom. Program 3 may allow noise reduction in addition to activation of directional microphones. Program 4 could be set to accommodate FM or perhaps a telecoil as discussed below.

Therefore, multiple programs allow flexibility to maximally process sounds in variable environments. In some advanced circuits, the programs may change automatically depending on the acoustic environment, i.e. adaptive processing. The hearing aid may essentially have only a single program, with multiple programmable attributes that are activated based on the hearing loss, the environment and the individual needs.

2) *Directional Microphones*

A very useful feature that should be considered is directional microphone technology. They allow an increase in the signal-to-noise ratio (SNR) which makes speech easier to hear. Basically, this technology allows sounds from the rear to be reduced relative to sounds from the front which is typically the location of the primary speaker. Because most children will be engaged in learning situations with information presented in front of them, it is highly desirable to reduce background noise through directional microphones. Hawkins and Yacullo (1984) have shown an increase in speech recognition of 25% when directional microphones were used compared to hearing aids with non-directional microphones. For young children and infants who may receive speech from a variety of speakers around them, parents may want the option to have two programs in the aid: a directional setting to focus on sounds from the front, and an omnidirectional setting to pick up sounds equally from all around. Recently, the option for "adaptive directional" microphones has become available. In essence, this involves automatic function of the directional microphone so that regardless of where the speaker is, in front or to the side, the microphone will focus on the speech and reduce the unwanted noise. [Several tutorials regarding the benefits of directional microphones are available at: *http://www.gennum.com/hip/front wave/index.html*]

3) *Compression*

Another feature common on most hearing aids is compression. This is a method of limiting the output of a hearing aid very quickly when a loud sound is presented so that the amplified sound remains comfortable with limited distortion. This can be thought of as a means of preventing sounds from becoming too loud, but doing so in a gradual way. A common analogy is a car approaching a stop sign that slows down several feet before rather than suddenly braking right at the sign. The sudden brake method is known as peak clipping where the intense portions of the amplified signal could be clipped and result in distortion.

There are many options for the compression settings and one that is commonly used is called Wide Dynamic Range Compression (WDRC). The goal of WDRC is to restore the range of loudness for the child such that soft sounds are perceived as soft, medium-level sounds are medium, and loud sounds are not too loud. Another feature related to compression in some digital hearing aids is the ability to set compression for many separate channels across the pitch range. This is helpful when a loud, low-pitched sound is heard while someone is speaking. An aid with multichannel compression can reduce the gain for the low-frequency sound, while maintaining audibility of the important speech cues in the higher frequencies.

4) *Noise Reduction Circuitry*

Most DSP hearing aids are designed with noise reduction circuitry. This may happen automatically or be chosen by the user in a specific program. The noise reduction circuit is designed to reduce the effects of the noise which is typically a repetitive, steady-state, low frequency signal, such as the noise made by a refrigerator. This is often accomplished based on the fluctuations of sound in the environment. DSP circuits are designed to recognize the fluctuations of speech versus the steady nature of noise. When the noise is detected, the DSP circuit reduces the gain for the noise while maintaining the gain for the higher-frequency speech cues. Research has shown that such circuits do provide benefits, particularly when combined with other noise reduction features such as directional microphones (Kuk, Kollofski, Brown, Melum, and Rosenthal, 1999).

5) *FM Compatibility*

Most BTE hearing aids are compatible with FM systems which allow for a significant improvement in speech recognition in noise, a highly desirable feature in school settings. The FM system is a short-range broadcasting system similar to an FM radio station, which has a much greater transmission range. The FM system consists of two main parts: the transmitter worn by the teacher, and the receiver worn by the child. By placing a microphone on the teacher and delivering this signal directly to the child, the problems of noise and distance from the speaker are dramatically reduced. Lewis et al. (2004) showed that the improvements in speech recognition in noise with an FM system were greater than with noise reduction circuitry in digital aids. There are three main ways in which the FM signal may be received in a BTE aid which include *direct audio input* (DAI), *T-coil* (see next section), and *internal FM receiver* in the BTE case. The FM receiver that is built into the BTE case is preferable because there are no external parts that can get lost. With DAI, the small FM receiver attaches to the aid via an "audio shoe" that slips onto the base of the aid. The switch settings on the BTE may need to be programmed so that the child can have the option for listening only to the teacher, and the option to listen to the teacher while hearing classmates nearby.

6) *T-coil Reception*

Another necessary feature in a hearing aid whether for children or adults is a T-coil, also known as telecoil, so that accommodations may be accessed in public places. T-coils are simply a coil of wire in the hearing aid that can be activated by a "T" switch on the hearing aid. If the T-coil is activated and the hearing aid is placed within a wire loop that produces an electromagnetic field, the hearing aid can pick up the transmitted signal. Although originally developed to improve reception of speech through a telephone, the most common use for children is in the classroom.

In some school districts, a T-coil is needed in the hearing aid to receive the signal from the FM system and greatly enhances reception of the teacher's voice. The signal from the FM transmitter worn by a teacher is sent to the FM receiver worn by the child. The signal is delivered to the hearing aid via a loop worn around the neck. The hearing aid must have a T-coil to pick up this enhanced signal. Devices with T-coils should have not only a "T" switch but also an "MT" switch which allows the microphone to remain active while the T-coil is functioning so that sounds can be received through the normal microphone pathway and the T-coil simultaneously. Hawkins (1984) has shown significant advantages in speech recognition in noise when using neckloop arrangements with FM systems. T-coils are also helpful in public places with induction loop systems. With the passage of the Americans with Disabilities Act in 1990 and efforts such as Loop America, more facilities are providing induction loop arrangements that are compatible with T-coils in personal hearing aids. [More information regarding the benefits of T-coils is available at:www.hearingloop.org]

7) *Child Appropriate Features*

There are at least three physical features that parents should explore that are particularly appropriate for children. A locking battery door removes the potential hazard of a young child swallowing a battery. The next feature is deactivation of the volume control. When this is done, the aid is preset to an optimal level and volume may be adjusted automatically if needed. The volume wheel can be rotated, but no change in sound occurs when the control is deactivated. This eliminates the concern that a child may increase the volume to harmful or subaudible levels.

The last feature to consider is the color of hearing aids. Just as children are frequently allowed to choose the color of their orthodontic retainer, they should be included in the decision regarding the color of their hearing aids. Color plays an important role in acceptance of hearing aids. If parents choose a bright color or one that can be color coordinated with clothing, people will more likely ask about the child's hearing loss and provide the opportunity for parents to discuss it openly in front of their child. This is in contrast to choosing a color or size so that it's not too obvious which sends the strong message that this is something to hide. If the child is taught to hide the hearing aids because it's a sign of weakness, they may develop low self-image and have negative reactions to amplification. Such a child is likely to reject the aids when encountering questions or hurtful comments from peers. Many manufacturers now have case covers that can be switched much like the covers of personal cell phones can be changed. A positive attitude toward amplification is considered paramount because if the child rejects hearing aids, then all the effort spent on choosing sophisticated features for acoustic processing of sound is of no value.

8) *One versus Two Hearing Aids*

When both ears can benefit from amplification, two hearing aids should always be considered. For children with a unilateral hearing loss, wearing a hearing aid on the impaired side or a system that picks up sound from that side and sends it to the good ear is often recommended. This helps to improve speech recognition when the speaker is on the impaired side. The optimal arrangement for children to gain access to auditory information is a binaural fitting (wearing two hearing aids). Stimulation of both auditory pathways contributes to normal brain development and facilitates speech and language development.

For children with bilateral hearing loss, there are four main reasons for wearing devices on each ear:
a) improvements in hearing soft sounds
b) understanding speech in noise
c) hearing speech equally well from speakers on either side
d) keeping both auditory pathways stimulated to prevent loss of neural connections.

Although energy arriving at each ear is processed through the auditory pathways on the respective sides, as the sound is transmitted to the brain, the excitation from one side crosses over and is combined with excitation from the opposite ear. It is the combination of excitation from each ear that results in the first three benefits of wearing two devices over just one.

The ability to hear soft sounds better with two aids compared to one is due to the stimulation of each ear combining to result in what is called binaural summation. Because the energy is summed, less gain is required from each hearing aid which results in longer battery life. Children with two hearing aids may receive about a 5 dB advantage in hearing sounds compared to wearing just one. Recall that decibels (dB) are units of sound depicted on the audiogram that are used to quantify how much a child can hear. The second reason for wearing two aids is that when noise arrives at two ears in certain ways, the actual interference of the noise (masking) can be reduced by the interaction of the acoustic stimulation at each side which is called *masking level difference.* Research has shown that persons with two hearing aids can hear about 20% more in noisy environments compared to just wearing one. It is also helpful to have two devices so that no matter what side a speaker is on, the speech can be received equally well. When only one hearing aid is worn and the speaker is standing opposite the side the hearing aid is worn, the sound must travel around the head to reach the hearing aid microphone. In this process, sound energy is lost and some of the important cues for speech understanding are not received. Finally, it's important to keep both ears stimulated so that the neural connections are maintained. Based on research with animals, it has been determined that lack of acoustic input to one side results in changes at the auditory cortex which may be irreversible (Robertson & Irvine, 1989).

9) *Feedback Reduction*

Hearing aid feedback is the whistling sound that occurs when amplified sound leaks from the hearing aid system and is re-amplified through the hearing aid microphone. Feedback is usually more annoying to others because often the child can't hear it. In advanced technology hearing aids, feedback reduction circuits have been incorporated to cancel feedback within the hearing aid very quickly, after it has been detected. If excessive feedback is present, the earmold may need to be remade and/or the hearing aid gain adjusted.

Hearing Aid Fitting

Following the audiogram, the results will be discussed and recommendations will be made with the parent(s). After the family has had time to review the information and explore options, the hearing aid fitting process may begin. After reviewing many of the considerations that impact selection of hearing aids, earmold impressions will be taken so that the proper style and features can be specifically made for the child. After examining the ears with an otoscope, the hearing care provider inserts a small sponge block. This is followed by molding material into the ear canal that stiffens but holds the shape of the ear when removed after about 15 minutes. Although the feeling of the material being inserted is unusual and it may seem uncomfortable, it is not painful. The child may be invited to bring a doll or stuffed animal that can be used for demonstration and/or for keeping hands "occupied." The impression is sent to a laboratory where the earmold is fabricated and returned in about one week.

To adjust the hearing aid precisely for a child's hearing loss and save time in the fitting process, the next step in fitting the hearing aid is to obtain what is called the *real-ear-to-coupler difference* (RECD). This is needed so that the sound of the hearing aid can be adjusted for the specific size of the child's ear. The output of hearing aids is measured in a metal coupler which is not the same size as the child's ear. Therefore, corrections are needed to account for this size difference. To measure the RECD, a small, flexible foam insert with a sound tube and a microphone tube is placed in the child's ear and the actual sound in the ear canal is measured when a specific sound is presented. Then the same sound is presented into a small metal coupler used to evaluate the output of hearing aids. The response is then compared to that obtained in the child's ear. The difference between the sound in the "real ear" and the sound in the "coupler" (RECD) is then used to preset the aid. This five-minute procedure facilitates the fitting process because the size and shape of a child's ear can affect the sound from the hearing aid and should be accounted for in the initial settings. For example, if the child has a very small ear canal, the sound from the hearing aid will not need to provide as high an intensity as it will for an older child with a larger ear canal. If the RECD measure cannot be done, predicted values can be used based on systematic research to record the RECD based on age of the child.

The options on hearing aids and price range will be discussed and parents can indicate preferences to guide the hearing care provider in selecting the hearing aid. The hearing care provider will preset the hearing aid before the child arrives based on the RECD and research that supports certain acoustic features for that type and degree of hearing loss (Seewald, Moodie, & Sinclair, 1999). Because hearing aids can be programmed for specific losses through the use of a computer, parents can often take home the hearing aid that is used in the evaluation.

At the next appointment, the earmold will be checked and the hearing aid will be tried for the first time. The hearing care provider may choose to first place the hearing aid on the parent or a doll for demonstration depending on the age of the child. After placing the aid on the child, there are several ways that the settings of the aid can be verified. The most accurate way is to measure the sound in the child's ear canal while wearing the aid through what is called real ear measures that take about five minutes per ear to complete. Through the use of a computer, the target acoustic response based on the child's hearing loss and age can be determined. The actual amplified sound level in the child's ear can be measured with a small, flexible probe tube placed along side the earmold while the hearing aid is in place. The target and the real ear response can be compared to determine if adjustments are needed in the acoustic output of the aid. The goal is for the actual sound measured in the child's ear canal to closely match the target for the amplified sound. In addition to the objective real ear measures, the child's response to sound will also be evaluated in the test booth.

Although many hearing aids have a two-year warranty which covers even accidental loss, variations in coverage as well as options for continuing coverage should be reviewed. Most states mandate a 30-day trial period with hearing aids so that parents may decide to return them for a refund, minus a small dispensing fee, if they believe it is not helpful for their child. If problems persist, the hearing care provider works with the family to find more suitable hearing aids perhaps with more desirable features. This may be a difficult decision because the child may just be learning to respond to sound or even keeping the hearing aids on at first. This adjustment could take longer than 30 days. In some cases, the 30-day trial can be extended through close communication with the hearing care provider.

Evaluation of Hearing Aid Benefit

At the initial fitting appointment, it is important to obtain some measure of the child's response to sound. Although the precise adjustments to amplification can be based on real-ear measures, the hearing care provider will need to confirm that the child is responding favorably. This is typically done by presenting speech through loudspeakers in the sound booth and finding the lowest intensity level that elicits a response. Aided soundfield responses to tones are often difficult to interpret because of advanced circuitry in hearing aids. The compression circuit may cause aided thresholds to indicate greater gain than is actually provided by the hearing aid for typical input levels analogous to conversational speech.

Input from teachers and/or caregivers may also be needed to evaluate the benefit of hearing aids for the child. A questionnaire may be used to document a child's performance with the hearing aid. One example, known as the Children's Outcome Worksheet (COW), allows for addressing situations specific to a given child from the perspectives of the parent, child and teacher. In addition, the educational audiologist at the child's school should be consulted, even if the child does not attend an organized class yet, so that any compatibility issues with FM systems provided by the school can be resolved during the 30-day trial. FM systems are provided in most educational settings for children with hearing loss to allow better reception of the teacher's voice as described later.

Orientation to the Hearing Aid Operation

At the hearing aid fitting, the hearing care provider will provide instruction on the care and use of hearing aids. Several topics may be included as summarized in Table 3-I. In addition to basic operation of the hearing aid, the parent will need guidance on the initial adjustment to them. Because hearing aids amplify new sounds for the child, it might take some time before meaning can be attached to the new sounds. These associations are developed as family members and therapists are pointing out sounds that are heard in the environment. This adjustment period may take as long as two to three months before the child consistently accepts the amplification for a whole day. Creative distractions may be needed at first, such as a new toy that may keep the child's hands occupied and thus not able to remove the hearing aids from the ears. Some hearing aid manufacturers provide children's books about wearing hearing aids and/or stuffed animals wearing hearing aids to help parents introduce amplification. At first, it may also be necessary to provide frequent breaks from wearing the aid. These breaks should be initiated by the parent removing them rather than the child. If there isn't a gradual acceptance of wearing hearing aids for longer time periods, there may be some cause for discomfort such as the physical fit of the earmold or the quality of the signal. Redness in the ear may be an indication of rubbing in a particular area and the need for an earmold modification or remake.

Parents will also need to practice inserting the hearing aids to learn the proper position. Even when the earmold is positioned properly, it may be difficult to keep the aid positioned on small ears. Suggestions to hold the aid in place include using hair tape found at beauty-supply stores and/or Huggie rings (*www.huggies.com*) from the hearing care provider. These rings fit around the child's ears and attach to the hearing aid by a thick rubber-band ring that fits around the body of each aid. When the earmold is not in proper position, there may be feedback, which is the loud squealing caused by amplified sound leaking back through the microphone and being re-amplified. This is often eliminated by proper positioning of the earmold. Feedback will occur as the child outgrows the earmolds. New earmolds are needed about every six months for children less than two years of age and annually thereafter until they're about eight or nine years old.

Table 3-I Options for personal FM Systems

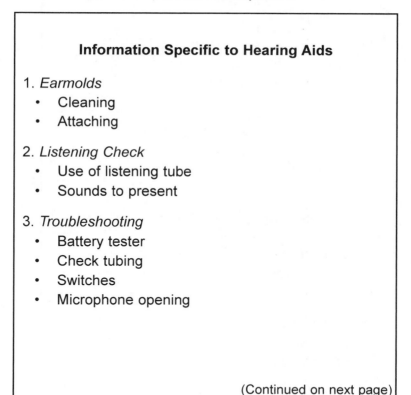

Information Specific to Hearing Aids

1. *Earmolds*
   - Cleaning
   - Attaching

2. *Listening Check*
   - Use of listening tube
   - Sounds to present

3. *Troubleshooting*
   - Battery tester
   - Check tubing
   - Switches
   - Microphone opening

(Continued on next page)

Table 3-I Options for personal FM Systems (Con't)

Information Regarding
Use of Cochlear Implants and Hearing Aids

1. *Batteries*
   - Checking the battery voltage
   - Insertion of the battery
   - Typical battery life

2. *Use*
   - Insertion and removal
   - Storage in Dri-Aid kit
   - Settings

3. *Care*
   - Protection from heat
   - Protection from moisture
   - Cleaning

4. *Possible Interface with FM System*
   - Receivers to consider
   - Transmitter options

Information Specific to Cochlear Implants

1. *Placement of External Components*
   - Speech processor
   - Coil

2. *Functioning Check*
   - Signal wand
   - Behavioral response

3. *Troubleshooting*
   - Battery tester
   - Charging batteries
   - Replace cords

4. *Protection against Electrostatic Charges*

Cochlear Implants

A cochlear implant is a surgically implanted device which provides electrical stimulation to the ear that the child can interpret as sound. The process of obtaining a cochlear implant is much more involved than that of receiving a hearing aid. The steps involved include the evaluation, the surgery, the activation and rehabilitation. As with hearing aids, significant aural rehabilitation is needed for the child to "learn to hear" through the implant. Children who are implanted very young, even at 12 months, have been successfully educated in regular classrooms in public schools and even use the telephone. It is very important to understand that despite many successful cochlear implant users, the exact outcome for any given individual cannot be accurately predicted. The particular characteristics of each child including the onset of the loss, mental abilities, communication experiences, ear anatomy, family involvement and communication therapy will altogether influence the success with the cochlear implant. The journey to developing communication through a cochlear implant will involve combined efforts of many people. Two important concepts for the parents of the child who receives a cochlear implant are 1) the willingness to embrace and commit to the use of oral skills, and 2) the necessity to enroll in an aural rehabilitation program to reinforce and strengthen auditory processing skills.

Evaluation for a Cochlear Implant

Many audiologists who fit cochlear implants are part of a team including the physician, a speech-language pathologist, psychologist, and/or an educator. It is a good idea for the parent(s) and the child to meet with each member of the team and for all team members to be in contact with each other to determine the best management protocol for the child. Cochlear implant teams are often associated with a medical center. Recently, cochlear implant specialty certification was offered by the American Board of Audiology (through the American Academy of Audiology) for those professionals providing service to users of cochlear implants. They must demonstrate competency by meeting requirements for education, audiology experience, direct patient contact hours, and a passing score on a standard examination. Parents may choose to seek out individuals with this specialty certification to ensure experience and knowledge in working with implants.

The criteria for candidacy include several factors related to the severity of one's hearing loss and the use of amplification. Children are considered candidates for cochlear implants when they do not receive benefit from powerful hearing aids after a trial period. Although generally these children have severe-to-profound hearing loss, some children with moderately-severe hearing loss may be considered candidates if they score less than 40% on a measure of speech recognition.

Another disorder for which a cochlear implant may be recommended is called *Auditory Neuropathy.* This refers to a lack of synchronization of the neural firings from the auditory nerve to the brain so that sound is not clear. Children with Auditory Neuropathy demonstrate abnormal results on an objective test of the brain's response to sound, the Auditory Brainstem Response or ABR test; yet they demonstrate a normal result on the cochlea's response to sound, the Otoacoustic Emission or OAE test. The cochlear implant has been helpful to children with Auditory Neuropathy because it helps to synchronize the neural response to sound through electrical stimulation of the auditory nerve and thereby increase the clarity of auditory information.

It's also important that a medical evaluation reveals adequate cochlear structure to receive the electrode array. Finally, the expectations of the child and/or family must be consistent with the potential benefits of the cochlear implant. They must realize that there will still be limitations to auditory performance and that benefit from cochlear implants develops over a considerable time period which varies across children. Some implant centers also require that the child be enrolled in an intervention program in which development of auditory skills is stressed. Regardless of this requirement, it will be necessary for the family to have a strong commitment to use oral skills and enroll in therapy focused on strengthening auditory processing of the new sounds the child will hear through the implant.

Cochlear implant technology today has allowed many children to identify words without prompting with the context or pictures, i.e. open-set speech recognition (Waltzman, Cohen, & Roland, 1999). However, just as with hearing aids, cochlear implants don't restore normal hearing and users are at a significant disadvantage when listening in noise (Battmer, Reid, & Lenarz, 1997; Fetterman and Domico, 2002; Hamzavi, Franz, Baumgartner, & Gsöettner, 2000; Schafer and Thibodeau, 2003). Parents will need to learn to control the acoustic environment for optimal communication with their child. The child, on the other hand, will need to learn how to listen and use the implant. Other technology may be interfaced with the cochlear implant to reduce unwanted interference in noisy environments. For example, with an FM system the speaker wears a microphone and the signal is transmitted directly into the cochlear implant speech processor.

After all the audiological testing is completed including speech-language and medical evaluations and a child has met candidacy criteria, the parents must select a cochlear implant device. Because there are only three cochlear implant manufacturers at the time of this writing, the decision of which device to use may be determined by what the surgeon and audiologist offer. Not all facilities have the equipment and expertise to work with all three manufacturers' products. In some cases, third-party reimbursement may determine the particular implant. However, when parents can choose one of the three manufacturers, one of the primary considerations should be the options for interfacing with hearing assistive technology such as an FM system to maximize benefits of the cochlear implant.

[More information regarding hearing loss and the process of getting a cochlear implant is provided in *the Parents Guide to Getting a Cochlear Implant* available at: *www.utdallas.edu/~thib*]

How Cochlear Implants Function

For the cochlear implant, there are four main components, two of which are external and two of which are implanted behind the child's ear. The external components include a speech processor and a transmission coil. The internal components include a receiver/stimulator and an electrode array. The sound enters the processor through a microphone, as shown in Figure 3-3. It is then converted into a series of pulses that correspond to the input signal and delivered to the external transmission coil. This coil which contains a magnet is held in place on the head by aligning it over another magnet that is surgically implanted in the bone behind the ear (the mastoid). The electrical pulses pass across the skin from the external coil to the internal receiver/stimulator coil and down to the electrode array that is surgically implanted into the cochlea, the inner portion of the ear. Auditory sensations are received from the pattern of pulses delivered to the nerve endings of the auditory nerve in the cochlea and interpreted by the child as meaningful sounds. Although batteries are needed for the externally-worn speech processor, there are no batteries for the internal portion.

Figure 3-3: Ear-Level cochlear implant with speech processor and external coil (left) and internal coil and electrode array (right).

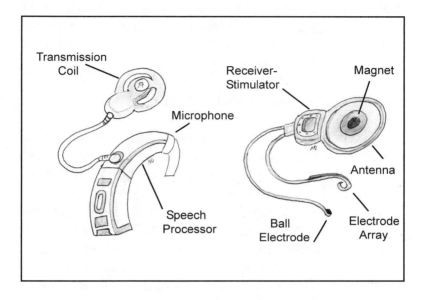

Cochlear Implant Surgery

When the implant is selected and a surgery date is scheduled, depending on the age of the child, several activities may be suggested to prepare the child and parents. These may include visits with other parents who have children with cochlear implants, adults with cochlear implants, and/or visits to the hospital to review the procedures and locations. The day of the surgery, the family will be with the child until the anesthesia is started at which time the child will be taken to the surgical area. In addition to shaving a small area of hair, a two-inch incision will be made behind the ear during surgery. After drilling a small circular area in the bone behind the ear, the internal coil is implanted in the bone behind the ear and the electrode array is inserted into the cochlea. After the operation, the doctor will talk with the family about the surgery and the child will be taken to the recovery area.

When the child begins to awaken after surgery, the family will stay with the child until they're allowed to go home, some even the same day. As with any surgery, there are risks which may include infection, facial nerve injury, anesthesia complications or leakage of cerebral spinal fluid. The risks should initially be explained by the doctor and reviewed again before surgery.

Activating the Cochlear Implant

The surgical site will need to heal for about three to four weeks before the external components can be added. During this time the child should continue to use the hearing aid on the non-implanted side. The day that the audiologist actually activates the cochlear implant processor for the first time is typically one of great excitement. At this time, the audiologist will add the external components and begin the process of determining the minimum current levels necessary for the child to hear and the maximum levels for comfort. Using a computer and interface to the speech processor, the stimulation levels will be adjusted for each electrode to develop what is called a *MAP* for the child. The child may play games like those used during the audiological evaluation or just play with toys while responses (such as eye-widening, searching for sound, smiles or possibly crying) are observed. It's not uncommon for a child to cry upon first hearing sound (as may happen with family members) because it is a new experience. They are not experiencing pain at this time, just an unfamiliar sensation that they'll learn to understand.

The initial MAPPING session may take as long as two hours until the proper stimulation is determined for each electrode. A procedure called *Neural Response Telemetry* may be used to help determine the MAP when there are no clear responses to sound. In response to stimulation provided by a computer, the activity of the auditory nerve is recorded and no response is needed from the child. If the child is implanted in both ears at once, of course the sessions may be longer or scheduled on consecutive days. If the child does not have a second implant, the recommendation is often made to continue wearing the hearing aid on the non-implanted ear. However, there should be another hearing aid evaluation to re-evaluate the settings on the hearing aid once the child is responding to the new sound provided by the implant on the opposite ear.

As with the initial hearing aid fitting, there will be much instruction regarding care and use of the cochlear implant which is summarized in the right side of Table 3-I. The parent may be provided handouts or instructional videos/DVDs to review all the information they receive at the initial fitting. Parents will try to keep the cochlear implant on the child as long as possible each day, even after the initial programming session. However, for some the new sound may be overwhelming at first and the wear time may need to be gradually increased. Likewise, the settings may be gradually increased each day when the child is first adjusting to the new sound. Just as with hearing aids, it may be difficult to keep the cochlear implant on at first. However, consistency in putting the implant back in place, if removed, sends a message that the device is not optional and very necessary.

There will be need to be close follow-up during the first months as the child learns to respond and understand the meanings of sound. During this time, the MAPPING may be changed to obtain optimal responses. As the brain is learning to interpret the new sound, the child may become more adjusted to louder sounds. If possible, the child's ability to understand speech will be determined each time in the sound-booth. The child's responses to individual frequencies may also be recorded on the audiogram. Re-evaluations will usually be conducted at least four times during the first year and annually thereafter unless changes in the child's responses require more frequent visits. The parents will be relied upon to make observations of the child's responses to help the audiologist determine the appropriateness of the settings. Often a journal may be kept of the sounds to which the child did or did not respond.

The fitting appointments are critical to the child's success. Whenever parents notice a lack of response or any change in response, the audiologist should be contacted. Sometimes devices may malfunction such that the child may still respond to sound, but he or she may not receive the specific stimulation for certain pitch sounds set in the initial MAP. When the implant is in need of repair, a loaner device should be provided if possible, so that the child is not without auditory stimulation.

Just like children who use hearing aids, children who receive cochlear implants will need intensive auditory therapy to learn to interpret sound in order to develop intelligible speech and acquire age-appropriate language skills. It is vital that the speech-language pathologist who provides this training be knowledgeable about cochlear implants so that any unexpected changes in the child's functioning can be communicated to the audiologist. Professionals with expertise in developing auditory communication may have certification as an Auditory Verbal Therapist, which means they have completed prescribed coursework, a national examination, and considerable practicum with children with hearing loss. Furthermore, this therapist often plays a significant role in monitoring the performance of the cochlear implant and guiding the family in expectations regarding auditory stimulation to facilitate communication development.

Hearing Assistive Technology

The use of hearing aids or cochlear implants does not restore hearing to normal. There could be many interfering effects on the sound before it reaches the microphone depending on the type of environment. Hearing assistive technology can reduce these unwanted effects. These devices are so important that a new tool has been suggested to complement the audiogram that audiologists and parents may consult as their child develops to determine what additional assistance may be needed. It has been proposed that in addition to the audiogram that represents the absolute hearing ability, the needs as represented on the TELEGRAM should also be considered to provide optimal communication assistance (Thibodeau, 2004b). As shown in Figure 3-4, this tool addresses several areas that can be facilitated by technology other than hearing aids. [A guide to hearing assistance technology (HAT) needs throughout the lifespan is provided in the HATs throughout Life brochure available at *www.utdallas.edu/~thib.*]

The first letter "T" refers to assistance that might be needed to communicate via the Telephone. Children with normal hearing begin listening to voices on the phone as early as one year of age usually when they're beginning to associate voices with family members. Simple methods to deliver the phone signal include using the speakerphone option or holding the phone handset over the microphone of the hearing aid while associating the voice with a picture of the person. As the child develops, more options may be considered, such as amplifiers that can be placed over the phone receiver, use of the T-switch on the hearing aid, or text-display phones. Many states have a program through which a free amplified phone is provided to individuals with hearing loss.

The second letter "E" refers to accommodations needed for access to Education or Employment activities. Typically, to overcome the noise and distance from the teacher in classroom settings, some type of FM system is used. The FM system includes a microphone and transmitter worn by the speaker through

Figure 3-4: The Telegram*

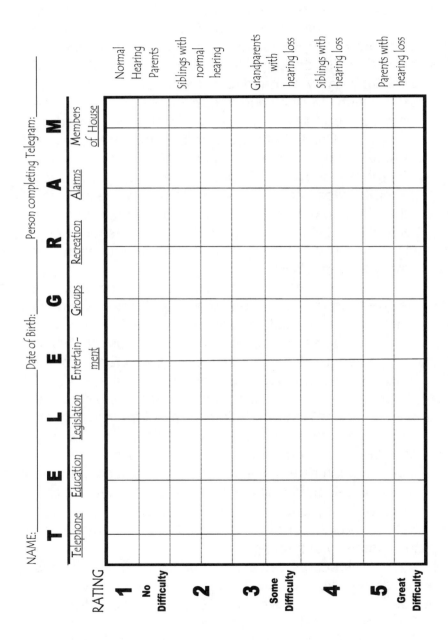

which the signal is sent via radio waves to the FM receiver worn by the person with hearing loss. The benefit of using this type of system is that a speaker's voice is received at a level above the background noise and remains constant regardless of distance. To illustrate how FM systems help reduce confusion created by background noise, a visual analogy is provided in Figure 3-5.

FIGURE 3-5: A visual analog to illustrate the effects of hearing loss and the benefits of FM Systems.

---

1) *Listening in Quiet at a soft level with normal hearing:*
I cdnuolt blveiee taht I cluod uesdnatnrd waht I was rdanieg. The aznamig pweor of the hmuan mind. Teh oredr of the ltteers in a wrod are not taht itnoamprt, the olny iprmoatnt tihng is taht the frist and lsat ltteer be in the rghit pclae. The rset can be a taotl mses and you can siltl raed it wouthit a porbelm. Tihs is bcuseae we do not raed ervey lteter by istlef, but raed the wrod as a wlohe.

2) *Listening in Quiet at a soft level with Hearing Loss:*
I wdreno if teh smae etfefc hpnpase fro plpeeo whti heraign lsos, btu tehri peocetpirn is aols hidnered by eenv further "rnearngirga" of ssodnu. Tehy otnef msis the lsta sndou. So it wlodu be enve hdrare.

3) *Listening in Noise with a Hearing Loss:*
Wtahxifzweptyrftosmilteauchraegnxinnnseoi?

4) *Listening in Noise with a Hearing Aid Alone:*

*Waht*x*difz***we***p***try***fto***m***s***slmitua***e***cdb***hraineg** *xi***nnsoie?**

5) *Listening in Noise with a Hearing Aid and FM System:*

*Waht*x*difz***we***p***tryfto***ms***slmituae***cdb***hraineg** *xi***nnnsoie?***

As discussed in the next chapter, the primary signal can get "smeared" with the noise so that there are no quiet pauses to help in segmenting the words. By placing a microphone on the speaker and transmitting the signal to the listener, the words are perceived more clearly because they're more intense than the background noise as show in the last section of Figure 3-5. Research with children using FM systems interfaced with cochlear implants has shown an average improvement in speech recognition of 26% for children (Schafer and Thibodeau, 2003) and 33% for adults (Schafer and Thibodeau, 2004).

Every child with hearing difficulties can potentially benefit from use of an FM system in an educational setting. Children served in public school will receive an FM system if they receive special services to address their hearing loss needs. An educational audiologist will be involved in selecting and setting the FM system for children in the schools. There are several factors that must be considered in selection of a system including other FM devices in use at the school, access to support personnel for troubleshooting, capabilities to interface with the child's hearing aids or cochlear implants and instructional arrangements. Whenever an FM system is selected that includes some modification to the personal hearing aid or cochlear implant, an evaluation is needed to ensure optimal settings on the equipment (Thibodeau, 2004a). During this evaluation, the output of the child's hearing aid will be compared to that obtained through the FM system using specialized hearing aid test equipment. Adjustments may be needed to the FM settings so that the acoustic characteristics of the FM system closely match that of the hearing aid. In particular, it is important that the maximum output of the two arrangements be matched and documented so there is no potential harm of overamplification by the FM system. [Demonstrations of the benefits of FM systems are provided in the audio demonstrations section of Educational Resources for Reducing Interference in Noisy Groups available at: *www.utdallas.edu/~thib.*]

Given that during a child's early years the parents are the primary educators, the family may consider purchasing an FM system for use in activities where noise may interfere with communication, such as large family gatherings, dining in restaurants, riding in a car or on outings to amusement parks, zoos and sporting events. Parents have reported that having a system for use at home resulted in enhancements to communication as they noted their child vocalizing more and they were reminded to provide vocal stimulation by wearing the microphone (Thibodeau and Schafer, 2002). In addition to providing an optimal signal through use of an FM system during the early years, the parent who wears the microphone on outings to the store or church is relaying to the child how important it is to receive acoustic information. When the parent is willing to wear a microphone and answer questions about its purpose, the child is learning to openly discuss hearing needs and accommodations.

The third letter in the TELEGRAM does not refer to a specific technology but to the topic of Legislation which is reviewed in the final chapter. In addition to assistive technology provided in educational settings, there is legislation which allows for assistive technology to be provided in many public facilities. Therefore, parents who purchase an FM system could check with children's programs for compatibility with their system. For example, the children's museum may provide tours using an FM system, but not provide equipment to interface with a child's specific cochlear implant. By inquiring prior to a visit, arrangements can possibly be made for compatibility to maximize communication.

The next three letters refer to Entertainment, Groups and Recreation. For a child these may all be the same activities such as birthday parties, ballet lessons, tumbling classes or sports activities. As manufacturers are beginning to include FM receivers within hearing aids so there are no special attachments, more families may begin to use the FM systems outside of the traditional educational settings.

The "A" in TELEGRAM represents the important accommodations that are needed for children to hear Alerting signals (such as doorbells, alarm clocks and smoke alarms). As with the telephone, parents will want to teach children the meaning of these signals throughout the developmental years. Assistive technology for alerting signals involves signaling the user via a light or vibratory signal. These devices range from simple, single unit items to more complex systems with transmitters and receivers. A simple system for signaling the presence of someone at the door is a vibration-sensitive device that is hung on the door. When someone knocks on the door, it has a light that flashes in the house. A more complex system could involve sensors connected around the house such as for the doorbell, the phone, the smoke alarm that transmit signals to a wristband that has areas that vibrate and illuminate specific to the auditory signals. In addition to providing these items in the home as a child develops, parents can ask for such accommodations as they travel and stay in hotels to continue teaching the value of technology in compensating for their hearing loss. It also alerts the travel industry of the necessity to accommodate their needs.

The final letter in TELEGRAM represents Members of the family that interact with the child. This is included to guide the audiologist in providing recommendations for optimal use of these systems. For example, if there is a large family with considerable conversation at the dinner table, a conference microphone may be suggested to enhance reception of the family members' interactions. If technology can be used to help connect the child with hearing loss with multiple family members, the language stimulation efforts will be multiplied as concepts are reinforced through incidental conversations as well as direct communication.

There are a variety of ways to obtain assistive technology. Many audiologists have a demonstration center in their office with devices available for trial. These may range from a full room set up like a living room to demonstrate devices available for use with the television or the telephone to a small cabinet containing a representative sample of devices. Many devices may also be purchased through the internet or at local electronics stores. Instruction regarding operation should be provided along with the opportunity for a 30-day trial. Because some are also capable of extremely high output sound pressure levels, these devices should be evaluated electroacoustically to verify appropriate settings for the child.

Conclusion

Parents who choose to communicate auditorily with their child with hearing loss will have many decisions to make. Information may be obtained from audiologists, speech-language pathologists, other parents, teachers, doctors and manufacturers. Regardless of the decision, the success of the child using the hearing aid and/or cochlear implant will depend in large part on the attitude with which the device is presented and treated within the family and community. Parents who openly acknowledge the device and encourage the child to show it to others or even participate in the process by wearing an FM transmitter, will be teaching the child very positive values that will create a foundation for using optimal technology throughout life. Digital technology to improve speech recognition in noise or bring high pitches within the range of hearing will be of limited value if the child believes that the hearing loss is something to hide. Parents will want to use the devices as tools to immerse their child into the world of sound, much like learning to walk allows a child to explore a whole new world.

With each discovery of sound, parents can share in the excitement that can continue into the teen years when the most rewarding auditory experiences might include listening to music on a CD or communicating over a cell phone. The choice may be for hearing aids, cochlear implants or a combination of the two. Regardless of the choice, parents who are involved in the process and encourage the consistent use of not only personal devices but also public assistive devices will be setting the stage for their child with hearing loss. On this stage their child will be more than an actor playing a supporting role, but an actor who is taking a lead role as model for others to cope with hearing loss.

References

Battmer, R.D., Reid, J.M. and Lenarz, T. (1997). Performance in quiet and noise with the Nucleus Spectra 22 and the Clarion CIS cochlear implant devices. Scandinavian Audiology 26, 240-246.

Fetterman, B.L. and Domico, E.H. (2002). Speech recognition in background noise of cochlear implant patients. Otolaryngology-Head and Neck Surgery 126, 257-263.

Hamzavi, J., Franz, P., Baumgartner, W.D. and Gsöettner, W. (2000). Hearing performance in noise of cochlear implant patients versus severely-profoundly hearing-impaired patients with hearing aids. Audiology 40, 26-31.

Hawkins D.B. (1984). Comparisons of speech recognition in noise by mildly-to-moderately hearing-impaired children using hearing aids and FM systems. Journal of Speech and Hearing Disorder 49, 409-418.

Hawkins, DB. and Yacullo, W. (1984). Signal-to-noise ratio advantage of binaural hearing aids and directional microphones under different levels of reverberation. Journal of Speech and Hearing Disorders

49,278-286.

Kuk, F.K., Kollofski, C., Brown, S., Melum, A., and Rosenthal, A. (1999). Use of a digital hearing aid with directional microphones in school-aged children. Journal of the American Academy of Audiology 10, 535-548.

Lewis, M.S., Crandell, C.C., Valente, M., and Horn, J.E. (2004). Speech perception in noise: directional microphones versus frequency modulation (FM) systems. Journal of the American Academy of Audiology 15, 426-439.

Schafer, E. and Thibodeau, L. (2003). Speech Recognition Performance of Children using Cochlear Implants and FM Systems. Journal of Educational Audiology 11, 15-26.

Schafer, E. and Thibodeau, L. (2004). Speech Recognition Abilities of Adults Using Cochlear Implants with FM Systems. Journal of the American Academy of Audiology 15, 678-691.

Seewald, R., Moodie, K.S., and Sinclair, S. (1999). Predictive validity of a procedure for pediatric hearing instrument fitting. American Journal of Audiology 8, 1-10.

Sininger, Y.S., Doyle, K.J., and Moore, J.K. (1999). The case for early identification of hearing loss in children. Auditory system development, experimental auditory deprivation, and development of speech perception and hearing. Pediatr Clin North Am 1,1-14.

Thibodeau, L. (2004a). Maximizing Communication via Hearing Assistance Technology: Plotting beyond the Audiogram! Special Issue: Assistive Listening Devices. Hearing Journal 57 (11), 25-32.

Thibodeau, L. (2004b). FM Systems: Terminology and Standardization. Proceedings from the International Conference on Achieving Clear Communication by Employing Sound Solutions (ACCESS) Conference. Chicago, IL.

Thibodeau, L. & Schafer, E. (2002). Issues to consider regarding use of FM systems with infants with hearing loss. ASHA Special Interest Division Newsletter, April, 18-21.

Waltzman, S.B., Cohen, N.L., and Roland, J.T. (1999). A comparison of the growth of open-set speech perception between the Nucleus 22 and Nucleus 24 cochlear implant systems. The American Journal of Otology 20, 435-441.

p

Chapter 4

Listening as a Gateway to Learning

Karen L. Anderson, Ph. D.

Dr. Anderson was an educational audiologist for 15 years, consulting with parents and teachers about the needs of children with hearing loss, managing amplification device wear, and providing aural habilitation services to children. She is the author or the co-author of the Screening Instrument For Targeting Educational Risk (SIFTER), Preschool SIFTER, Secondary SIFTER, Listening Inventory For Education (LIFE), Children's Home Inventory of Listening Difficulty (CHILD), Early Listening Function (ELF) test. Her writing and research has focused on the listening needs of children with hearing loss in the regular classroom. She participated on the ANSI 12 Work Group that developed the 2002 Acoustical Performance Criteria, Design Requirements, and Guidelines for Schools and is the 2003 recipient of the Educational Audiology Association's Fred Berg Award.

Dr. Anderson currently serves as the early hearing loss detection and intervention audiology consultant and coordinator of early intervention services for children with hearing loss in the State of Florida.

Due to the success of newborn hearing screening and early identification of hearing loss, parents now have the opportunity to spend countless hours arranging the world of a child with hearing loss so that he or she can learn language from listening in everyday situations. During early intervention services, parents come to understand that the child's sensory devices, whether they be high technology hearing aids or cochlear implants, are the lifeline that the child uses to learn language and the meaning of the many sounds that provide important information. Parents typically become aware of the size of their child's listening bubble—how close the parent needs to be for the child to be able to detect a sound and the distance needed for the child to really hear the parent's speech well enough to understand what is said (see Figure 4-1).

In the early years of the child's life the parents also develop an awareness that background noise in the car, grocery store or fast-food restaurant causes the child's listening bubble to be much smaller and conversation much more challenging. After all of the many hours of interacting with the child—talking, teaching, listening and learning—parents can be proud of their son's or daughter's hard earned success as a communicator. This success is a credit to early dedication to the child's future and to providing the child with a rich listening and language environment.

During the first few years of life many children with hearing loss master repeating the Ling sounds (/oo/, /ah/, /ee/, /sh/, /s/, /m/) as the parents and children work together to check the functionality of the hearing aids or cochlear implants. The child may have become very dependable, reporting to the parent when a problem occurs with a hearing aid or the speech processor on the implant. This is evidence that the child can recognize that malfunctioning technology is a break or weakness in the lifeline to a world of sound. Although some children may rely on attending to visual cues or sign language, most children who are identified with hearing loss shortly after birth will develop skills to allow them to learn and monitor their world through what they hear with amplification.

Children identified with hearing loss today can experience a future that is much brighter than most children with hearing loss from previous decades. Early hearing loss detection, early hearing aid fitting, appropriate early intervention services and truly

Figure 4-1: Representation of the *Listening Bubble* concept
—Effect of hearing loss on distance listening.

Not in Range

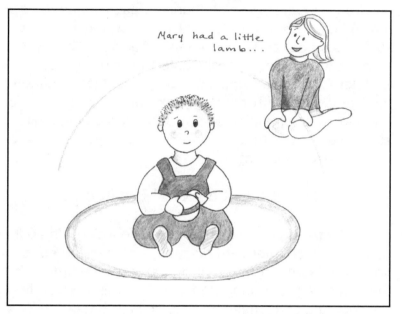

In Range and Listening

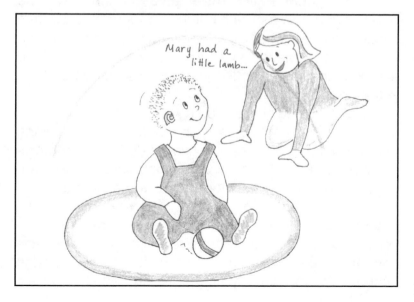

involved parents communicating effectively and frequently have been found to be the four keys to preventing language and learning delays in children with hearing loss. The result is an increasing number of children with all degrees of hearing loss who have normal or near-normal language skills by the time they start preschool or kindergarten. After all of the work, time, care and expense invested during infancy and "toddlerhood," many parents begin to feel confident that their child with hearing loss has learned what is needed to communicate, socialize and be educated side-by-side with other children of his or her age who do not have a hearing loss.

Entering the Educational Environment

Listening is a vital gateway to learning. The purpose of this chapter is to discuss factors in the educational environment that can be barriers to learning for the child with hearing loss. This chapter will first describe the challenges that the child with hearing loss will face in perceiving speech as clearly as possible in a school setting. These different issues interrelate to create a unique ability to perceive speech and cope with hearing loss for each child. Although the mounting challenges can seem overwhelming and depressing, solutions or a means to address a child's intrinsic and extrinsic challenges to listening will be described later in the chapter.

Successfully developing communication skills by age 3 has resulted in many children with hearing loss spending their preschool years (3 to 5) in community preschool settings. In preschool, children are typically provided a variety of structured activities. However, there's one constant when young children gather together—noise. In these early learning situations, the confidence many parents feel in their child's communication skills can begin to falter. This change occurs because when young children gather together, noise and its extra challenge to listening enters the scene.

- *Sam's teacher says that he plays alone most of the time but I know he loves it when Robert comes to our house and they play together so well!*
- *He is always so exhausted when he comes home from preschool.*
- *Jasmine's teacher said that she wasn't following directions. I know that Jasmine knows the words the teacher is using and she usually tries so hard to please.*
- *Jamal has always been so chatty with us at home. He and his sister play house together and build with blocks. In preschool his teacher said he hardly says a word and just watches the other children as they play.*
- *He pushed a child down! We've always taught him to share and to ask for toys and today his teacher said Travis just pushed another little boy down and pulled a toy out of his hands!*
- *The teacher says that Maria often acts as though she is in her own little world.*

Noise as a Barrier to Learning

The American National Standard 2002 Acoustical Performance Criteria, Design Requirements and Guidelines for Schools refers to the barrier that noise poses in the classroom to a student with hearing loss as being just as significant as a high threshold is to a child in a wheelchair who wants to join his or her peers in accessing regular instruction. With little effort people with normal hearing can mentally block out or ignore the noise around them and focus on listening to what someone is saying. This is a skill learned without conscious effort as people with normal hearing are exposed to different communication situations in background noise.

High technology hearing aids and well-mapped cochlear implants process all types of sound. Unfortunately, background noise and the desired speech signal are meshed together in an acoustic package that is then delivered to the child's brain. All young children have some difficulty processing speech when background noise is also present, but the child with hearing loss is at a much greater disadvantage. Even adults with hearing loss who have worn hearing aids since their youth and spent countless hours in all types of listening situations do not develop the ability to selectively listen through noise as well as people who are not hearing impaired. In other words, noise is a critical issue for a student with hearing loss who needs to be able to access verbal instruction in a classroom setting. It's very important to consider how much of a barrier the acoustic environment poses to the child as he or she strives to perceive what is said by the teacher and other students.

Fragility of the Speech Signal

Understanding hearing loss is about more than being able to read an audiogram. What is the child's ability to understand words in quiet (word discrimination score)? This will change as the level of background noise increases. Hearing aids and cochlear implants don't restore normal hearing like glasses can restore normal vision. Some speech sounds are harder to hear because the phonemes vary in their level of loudness. Consider the word "thaw." The end sound /aw/ is a loud low frequency (pitch) speech sound. Compare this to the phoneme /th/ as in the word "with," which is a quiet high frequency speech sound. Low frequency speech sounds just naturally tend to be louder than high frequency sounds. The average loudness (sound pressure level in decibels [dB] of conversational speech) is about 45 dB, but this number represents the range of loudness of speech sounds. Therefore, some phonemes in conversation can be about 60 dB and other parts of speech can be as quiet as 30 dB.

Many children have hearing loss greater in high frequencies than in low frequencies. Children with cochlear implants hear all the pitches at about the same level but they tend to hear the high frequency sounds (/s/, /th/, /ch/) better than most children with hearing aids. Knowing the configuration of the child's hearing loss (meaning how well they hear the different pitches relative to the whole pitch range) when they're wearing their hearing aids or cochlear implants is important to know as his or her ability to perceive speech in any setting including the classroom is considered. If a child has substantial hearing loss in the high frequencies, then the fact that these high pitch sounds are quieter than low pitch sounds makes the challenge of listening to quiet speech or to speech in noise even more difficult.

Even for people with normal hearing it's not uncommon during daily conversation in a busy household or other active settings to "hear" that someone is talking but to not be able to understand everything that was said. This is because the softer speech sounds were not heard or were detected by the listener but were not loud enough to really be understood. Teachers of course talk louder than conversational speech when providing verbal instruction. The average loudness of a teacher's voice while instructing is 60 dB, with the loudness of speech sounds ranging from 45 to 75 dB. In order to perceive all of what the teacher said (to access verbal instruction), a listener would need to be able to hear the whole 30 decibel range of loudness of speech, not just the louder speech sounds.

Figure 4-2: Loudness range of some quieter and louder speech sounds in relation to loudness of background noise.

Signal-to-noise ratio +15 dB
Speech sounds all fully audible

Signal-to-noise ratio +6 dB. Louder vowels and parts of consonants audible.

30 dB speech signal range (45-75 dB) from quiet sounds (s, f) to loudest (oo, ay)

Signal-to-noise ratio 0 dB. Noise competes with hearing speech, especially quieter consonants.

oo ee ay i
m d b
sh ch s f t th

Typical loudness of background noise in classrooms is 60 dB (when little attention to room acoustics is given)

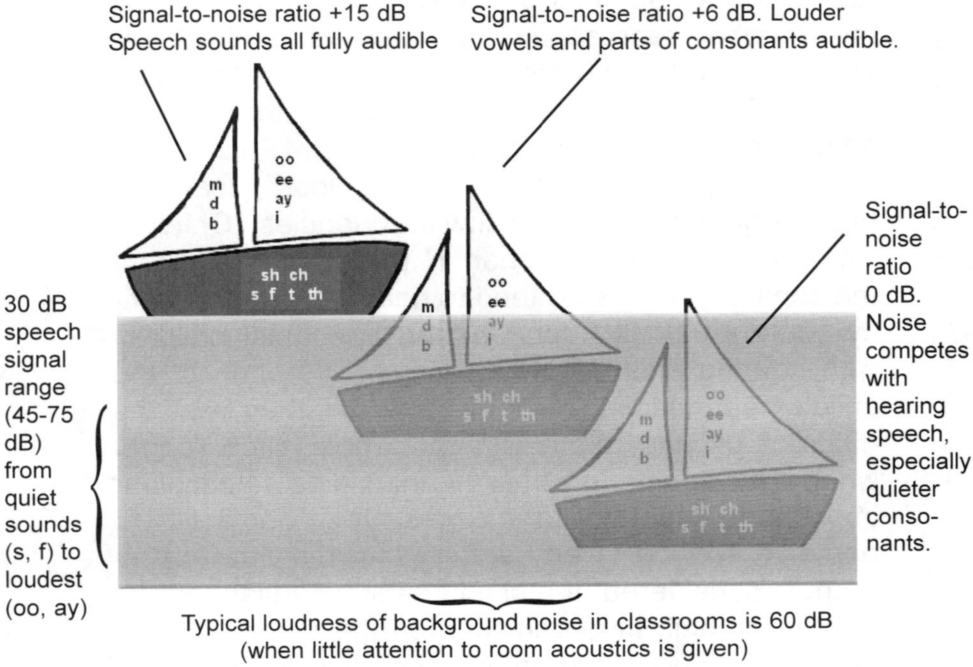

Figure 4-2 illustrates how the loudness of speech sounds varies over time from 45 dB to 75 dB, with the average level of the teacher's voice being 60 dB. The softer speech sounds (in the 45-60 dB portion of the speech signal) will mostly be high frequency consonants (such as /f/, /s/, /th/, /p/) or high frequency components of vowels (such as /i/ in bit). The louder speech sounds (in the 60-75 dB portion of the speech signal) will most likely be low frequency consonants (such as /d/, /m/) or most of the vowel sounds such as /ay/, /oo/, /aw/). When background noise is present it can interfere with just the quieter sounds of speech or all of the sounds of speech.

As illustrated in Figure 4-2, the speech signal that averages 15 dB above background noise will be loud enough to be heard over the noise. When a desired auditory signal is louder than an undesired auditory signal, like noise, this relationship is expressed as the signal-to-noise ratio, or S/N. Therefore, a speech signal 15 dB louder than the rumble of the room ventilation system would be described as having a +15 dB S/N. When the teacher's voice and the background noise is the same loudness, the quieter her words, especially the higher frequency portions of her speech will be buried by the background noise. This would be a 0 dB S/N signal – the speech and noise have equal loudness and therefore no (zero) difference. With 0 dB S/N the student might perceive that speech is occurring, but will have difficulty perceiving sounds like /s/ and /f/ and the quick unstressed parts of speech like word endings. Words like /cap/, /cat/ and /calf/ can get confused. That is, the /a/ vowel sound can be perceived, but the word beginnings and endings can be lost in a sea of noise. Speechreading (lipreading) when the teacher is talking will help when parts of words are not clearly heard, but it's not always possible to see the teacher's face and many of the speech sounds look the same on the lips (for example, /p/ and /b/, or /t/ and /d/).

Figure 4-3 illustrates a visual analogy of loudness, clarity and ease of recognizing speech sounds in

Figure 4-3: Visual analogy illustrating loudness, clarity and ease of recognizing speech sounds in different loudness levels speech over background noise.

I see some beautiful flowers.	+20 dB
Big dogs can be dangerous.	+15
I like to go to school.	+10
It is lunch time soon.	+5
Walk to the library now.	0
Your brother is not here.	-5

different loudness levels of speech over background noise. The range of loudness of different speech sounds means that the person with hearing loss typically misses fragments of speech (for example, /f/, /s/, /t/ sounds). Also, because normal hearing ability is not restored by hearing aids or cochlear implants, persons with hearing loss typically perceive speech at a quieter loudness than those with normal hearing. In other words, speech is both fragmented and quieter when perceived by the listener with hearing loss. Because of these factors, children with hearing loss need a bit more time to process the parts of speech they hear. To use an analogy of putting together a picture puzzle, they are continuously trying to figure out what the picture is when they do not have all of the pieces. Depending on the child's hearing loss, even when the room is quiet and the child is rested and motivated to hear the entire message, the equivalent of only 80 pieces of a 100-piece puzzle may be perceived (see Figure 4-4a).

In addition to fragmentation of the message because some sounds cannot be made audible due to the level of hearing loss, there are times in which moderate to severe hearing loss (about 60 dB and above) can cause sounds to be "mistuned" so that they're not interpreted as the correct frequency. This could be compared to having a 100-piece puzzle with 20 pieces missing. Ten of the twenty pieces fit into place, but these pieces do not have the right picture. If the acoustics in the learning environment further limit the amount of information clearly heard, a child may perceive only 60 of the 100 pieces (see Figure 4-4b). It may be very difficult and require much effort to figure out the big picture on an ongoing basis to continually pick up the pieces and try to make sense of them. The easier the picture puzzle (information the child already knows), the easier it will be for the child to figure out the full message. The more complex and detailed picture of the puzzle (new concept, vocabulary in a new

Figure 4-4a: Representation of fragmented speech due to hearing loss; puzzle analogy represents an 80% word discrimination score.

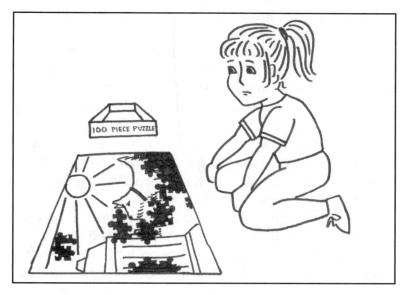

Figure 4-4b: Representation of fragmented speech due to hearing loss; puzzle analogy to represent a 60% word discrimination score.

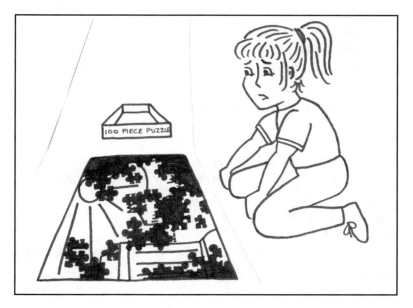

unit of study), the greater the chance that the information will not be fully understood.

The varying loudness of speech sounds that occur in a 30 dB range and the relation of the loudness range to high and low frequency sounds becomes especially important when we consider a student listening to a teacher or his or her classmates in the typical background noise present in a classroom. In a quiet setting, successful auditory learners with hearing loss have developed skills to really attend to what they're able to hear and combine this information with their knowledge of language and the context of the topic being discussed. They can achieve fair, good or even excellent understanding of speech.

When there's noise present, the quieter or less intense parts of speech are easily covered up by the unwanted sound. The phenomenon when one sound covers up another sound is called *masking*. Just as when a person wears a mask over his face it makes it difficult to recognize who they are, when background noise masks part of the teacher's voice it can make it difficult for the students to fully recognize what was said. The key to how easy it is to recognize a person's face, or the different sounds of speech, relies on how much of a face or the speech signal is really masked. Sources of school noise can be from the classroom itself (e.g., the ventilation system, child-generated noises, and noise from furniture or feet moving). Noise can also be from sources internal to the school but outside the classroom (e.g., the voice of the teacher in the adjacent room being transmitted through the wall or noise from busy hallways) or even from outside of the school building (e.g., playground noise, airplanes overhead, local construction or traffic noises). Any noise, regardless of the source, can cause interference to perception of speech.

As was previously mentioned, persons with hearing loss typically do not perceive high frequency sounds as well as those with normal hearing, thus making the effects of background noise on speech discrimination even more pronounced. Listeners with cochlear implants typically perceive high frequency speech sounds better than children who wear hearing aids but they will still perceive speech at a quieter level than people with normal hearing and continue to be very vulnerable to difficulty perceiving the speech signal when it's in competition with background noise.

To further illustrate this concept, here's an example of a direction given by a teacher: *"Please get out your math book and turn to page two sixty-seven."* An example of receiving the same information in quiet with a high frequency hearing loss, might be *"Leaz ge ou your ma boo an urn oo age oo ixie en."* An example of perceiving this information with high frequency hearing loss while listening in noise might be: *"Ee e ou or a oo an ur oo a oo iee en."*

Dynamics of Classroom Listening

Two other factors that complicate how children perceive verbal instruction in the classroom are their distance from the teacher and changes in the loudness of the teacher's voice during the day. Parents and teachers can easily notice that if a child with hearing loss is at some distance, he or she will be less likely to respond to speech, especially if noise is present from a busy fast-food restaurant or other noisy setting. Teachers typically move throughout the classroom as they teach and provide instructions. Therefore, they may be close to the student sometimes and far away at other times. Also, teachers change the loudness of their voice throughout the day in response to background noise level, emotional intensity and fatigue. As a result, the loudness of the teacher's speech relative to the noise (S/N) is constantly varying even if the child is always seated at the front of the classroom. Refer to http://www.voiceacademy.org for more information on how classroom acoustics can affect teacher voices and student listening. This constantly varying S/N is the reason why merely seating the child close to the teacher will be inadequate to meet the child's speech perception needs in a typical classroom setting. Preferential seating is not enough!

The relationship between the S/N and the distance from the teacher is illustrated in Figure 4-5. The level of background (ambient) noise in an occupied

Figure 4-5: Speech-to-Noise ratio as a function of distance in a room with 60 dB SPL ambient noise.

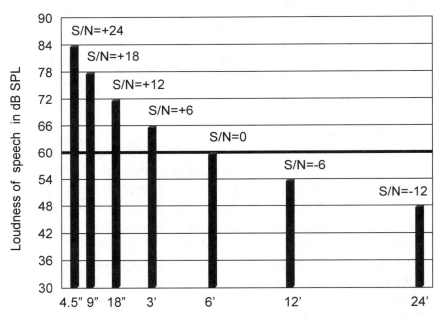

Distance of the child's ears or the teacher's microphone from the teacher's lips. [Adapted from Nabelek and Nabelek, 1985]

classroom can be 60 dB. If you will remember, the typical vocal loudness of the teacher is also 60 dB sound pressure level (SPL). Both the loudness of the teacher's voice and the background noise vary continuously resulting in periods in which the S/N may be relatively favorable (i.e., +10 S/N) to unfavorable (i.e., -6 S/N). A signal-to-noise ratio of +6 to -6 is not enough to bring all of the speech sounds out of the sea of noise (see Figure 4-2).

Most classrooms have background noise levels that result in a range of S/N occurring from -6 dB to +10 dB. Changes in S/N vary from moment to moment throughout the day. Even children seated close to the front row may be 6 to 12 feet from the teacher as she moves about the front of the room. As was shown in Figure 4-2, in order for the entire speech signal to be above the background noise the S/N must be +15 dB (this assumes no benefit from early reflected sound). Children with hearing loss, because they typically don't perceive speech as loudly or as completely as people with normal hearing, require a S/N even greater than +15 dB if they're to truly have equal access to verbal instruction.

The loudness of the teacher's voice is also an important factor that needs to be taken into account when considering S/N. Some teachers speak loudly, others have quieter voices. Classrooms with inappropriate levels of background noise require a teacher to raise the loudness of her voice for hours each day. Reducing background noise in a classroom to an appropriate level is an obvious way to try to achieve a +15 S/N. Unless the S/N ratio for the teacher's voice is increased by reducing the background noise or by applying S/N enhancing technology individually (e.g., personal FM system) for children with hearing loss, the S/N level present in a classroom will be both inconsistent and insufficient to meet the listening needs of the child with hearing loss.

If a classroom has many hard surfaces, listening becomes even more difficult because the hard surfaces reflect the sound and create what is called *reverberation.* Reverberation is sometimes called the echo in the room, but it's actually the length of time the sound continues to be heard as it's reflected off hard surfaces in the room. Think of a classroom as a 6-sided box with each of the sides being a surface covered with materials that reflect sound. The larger the surfaces in the room that are hard (vinyl floor, windows, cement block walls, painted or poor quality acoustic tile ceilings), the longer the sound reflections will last as they bounce from side to side of the box. Just as background noise serves to mask (cover up) the quieter parts of the speech signal, reverberation smears the direct signal of the teacher's voice with overlapping reflections of sound. Remember the visual analogy of this phenomenon illustrated in Figure 4-3? Another way to consider the effects of reverberation is to think of the picture puzzle analogy with the same pieces missing, but the lines of the picture have become blurred making the picture even more difficult to distinguish.

The key thing to remember for children with hearing loss is that they'll be able to use their available hearing to the best advantage in a room that has many soft surfaces, like carpeting, acoustic wall panels and drapes, rather than in a room with hard surfaces like shiny painted walls, vinyl flooring and ceiling tile with little texture or depth. Acoustic wall panels can be added to a room as can carpeting, or replacing ceiling tiles. Adding drapes, plants or tapestry wall hangings won't be enough to offset the sound reflections caused by reflective flooring and walls.

The reverberation time (RT) refers to how many seconds it takes for a loud sound (like a hand clap) to fully decay (dissipate) by 60 dB SPL. Large reverberant rooms like gymnasiums may have a RT of one to two seconds or more. Smaller quiet spaces like a fully furnished living room with carpet and upholstered furniture may have an RT of 0.3 to 0.4 seconds. Some sound reflection is necessary to reinforce the primary signal and allow it to be perceived easily. For example, it's easier to clearly hear someone when you're standing 12 feet away in an enclosed room than when you are standing outside 12 feet away where no sound reflections reinforce the signal. So a little reverberation is a good thing but too much reverberation will cause smearing of speech sounds and will actually add to the background noise level.

How much is too much? National standards for acoustics in learning environments (2002) recommend that RT be no more than 0.6 seconds. For the best perception of speech sounds without smearing, the person with hearing loss requires a RT of 0.3 – 0.4 seconds. Reverberation time is measured when a room is unoccupied. The presence of children also serves to dampen sound, therefore, when 20-30 students are present, a classroom with a 0.6 RT in daily listening may actually have 0.5 RT. Unfortunately, less than 1/3 of classrooms have reverberation levels of 0.6 seconds or less (Crandell and Smaldino, 1994) with actual classroom reverberation times ranging from 0.35 to 1.2 seconds. It is critical to understand that when sound is reflected in a classroom for a prolonged time (more than 0.6 seconds), this will also add to the overall background noise level in the classroom. Any classroom that's too reverberant will also have a noise problem because of the prolonged sound reflections.

It was mentioned earlier that perceiving speech becomes more difficult when distance increases. Reverberation adds to this problem. When a child is within a critical distance for listening, the child is close enough to the teacher for speech to travel directly from the teacher's mouth to the child's ears with minimal sound reflections. There's a formula for determining the exact critical distance based on the size of a room, but in typically-sized classrooms the critical distance is within less than ten feet of the teacher. When there is excessive reverberation, the critical distance shrinks, sometimes to only a few feet. In typically noisy, reverberant classrooms of average size even children who are preferentially seated are outside of the critical distance for listening.

To summarize, reverberation smears speech clarity (see Figure 4-6), prolongation of sound due to

Figure 4-6: Representation of smeared speech clarity due to hearing loss.

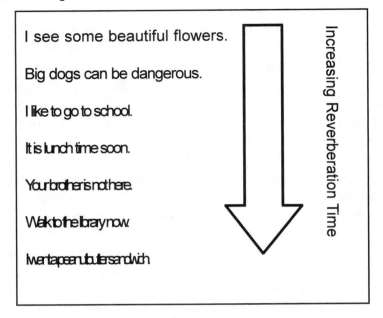

excessive reflections adds to the noise level in the classroom, and the critical distance for listening shortens as reverberation time increases. When we consider how much of a barrier acoustics is to learning in a classroom we need to consider:

- the background noise;
- the reverberation time;
- the typical vocal loudness of the teacher; and
- the child's distance from the teacher.

Of these four phenomena, all but reverberation are continuously being varied throughout the day in a typically dynamic learning environment.

The Work of Understanding Speech

Children with hearing loss usually have to learn with two challenges that children with normal hearing rarely experience: gaps in language and in listening. Even highly successful children with hearing loss are at risk for having some gaps in vocabulary and world knowledge. They miss more incidental language than their normal hearing peers because they're not as able to listen at a distance or passively overhear speech. Add to this the typical traits of speech fragmentation and perceiving speech at a quieter loudness that occur for most listeners with hearing loss, even when they use the latest technology (hearing aids or cochlear implant). These two factors already pose a challenge to learning, and now also add to that the negative effects of the acoustic conditions in the learning environment. Language gaps, listening gaps, and poor classroom acoustics work together to effect how well children with hearing loss are able to perceive the entire speech signal during verbal instruction in the typical classroom. These factors can further effect the child's development of phonemic awareness that is important for early reading skills and may contribute to syntax (grammar) deficiencies in writing. Output depends on input. The more the speech signal is fragmented, diminished, and smeared the greater the level of these effects on the outputs of language, reading, writing and social communication.

Listening is difficult when there are distractions. Visual or auditory distracters are present in every classroom. This could be the frequent sniffling of an allergic student two rows behind the child with hearing loss, a fluttering mobile hanging from the ceiling that catches the eye, laughter from the next room, etc. For all students, distractions can interfere with attention, thereby breaking the child's focus on listening, listening, listening. Distractions plus the other challenging factors that have been discussed result in the child needing to work harder as he or she tries to learn at the same rate and to the same level of understanding as classmates. In other words, the student with hearing loss must put forth more effort to actively perceive the verbal instruction that their peers with normal hearing passively perceive with little effort. This extra effort must be applied to every communication exchange with peers and every period of direct instruction as the teacher moves about the room, including effort toward understanding other children's responses during class discussions. It's not surprising that children with hearing loss are frequently exhausted at the end of the school day!

Teachers often comment that their students with hearing loss are not paying attention, that they miss directions, and that they allow themselves to become distracted easily. Making sure teachers have a good understanding of the effects of hearing loss on speech perception is necessary for them to understand why children with hearing loss may appear more inattentive than their peers with normal hearing. Parents can advocate and provide assistance to school staff to assist them in understanding the child's unique listening needs and what they require to function optimally in school. Selecting teachers who provide a consistent structure that the child can learn to depend on when they do not hear completely, teachers who have voices that project well over the classroom (versus being soft spoken), and teachers who are willing to be flexible and adjust as necessary to meet the child's listening needs will go a long way in setting up the child for a successful academic year.

Children who have hearing loss who were very successful language users and listeners upon entry into school at age 3 or 5 must work very hard as they become older to compete with children in their classes who don't have their same listening challenges. Indeed, it is predictable that without special accommodations (e.g., appropriate acoustics, FM equipment, seating, instruction checks) and/or support (e.g., speech language pathologist, teacher of the hearing impaired), children with hearing loss will experience a widening gap in their understanding of language, academics, social interactions and the ability to comprehend complex information because of their challenge in perceiving verbal instruction in the typical classroom.

Addressing Challenges or Barriers When Listening to Learn

1. Hearing loss causes a reduced "listening bubble" that is improved by hearing aids or cochlear implants but normal hearing is not restored.

2. Child misses some of the communication naturally occurring in their environment but beyond their "listening bubble."

3. The resulting gaps in language or world knowledge may be minimal to substantial.

4. Speech may be perceived with some sounds missing (i.e. high frequency consonants).

5. Hearing aids or cochlear implants deliver speech at a quieter loudness than what is typically heard by persons with normal hearing.

6. Ability to attend to verbal instruction varies over time with auditory and visual distractions, level of fatigue and interest.

7. When the speech puzzle is incomplete and smeared, the high pitch rapid speech of classmates can be incompletely heard and peer relationships may be affected.

8. Teacher vocal loudness, distance, and background noise change continuously.

9. Acoustic energy of speech decreases the farther away the child is from the teacher.

10. Background noise covers up quieter parts of speech.

11. Reverberation affects clarity of the perception of speech by smearing sounds, adding noise due to prolonged sound reflections and shortening the critical distance for listening.

12. When more effort is needed to perceive speech less energy is available to meaningfully comprehend what has been said and achievement is affected.

As previously described, there are many challenges or barriers to listening that often occur for the child with hearing loss who is listening to learn in a typical classroom. Children are amazingly resilient and adaptable. Learning does occur for children with hearing loss, especially when the educational system accommodates the child's difficulties perceiving verbal communication in the classroom. We can address barriers to learning. Teachers can become aware of the effects of the day-to-day challenges to each child's ability to learn in a typical educational environment.

Let's break down the twelve challenges into two groups. The first five of twelve challenges from the previous list occur within the child and the remaining seven are challenges within the learning environment. Factors within the child interact with environmental factors to produce unique learning characteristics. Although the child factors are of great importance and deserve careful consideration, this chapter will serve to provide only a cursory mention of some of the issues.

Addressing Challenges within the Child

Challenges within the child relate specifically to the child's degree of hearing loss, additional learning difficulties, success with amplification, and his or her level of school achievement compared with classmates who have normal hearing.

1. Hearing aids or cochlear implants improve the ability of the child to perceive sound but don't restore normal hearing. Therefore, even when the best personal hearing devices are worn, a child with hearing loss will continue to have a smaller 'listening bubble' as compared to normal hearing peers.

2. The smaller listening bubble will result in the child having decreased opportunities to perceive naturally occurring communication that goes on every day in

many situations. With appropriate early intervention to teach parents how to communicate and use language effectively from infancy, many children with hearing loss may have language levels that are equivalent or close approximations to the average language levels of peers with normal hearing when they enter school. In the range of cultural, ethnic and economic diversity in our present society, children come to school with variations in world knowledge and language understanding.

3. Gaps in language understanding will only grow if the parents, teacher and other school staff are not fully aware and diligent in preventing language delays. If the child has identifiable language deficits, then he or she can benefit from the services of a speech-language pathologist working with the classroom teacher to focus on language skills. Parents will need to do their part to help their child's continued language development at home. All children need to develop a questioning attitude about unfamiliar words, recognizing when they come across a new word, and using context and other skills to figure out what the new word may mean. A child with hearing loss who routinely may hear only parts of words will have more difficulty recognizing when a word may be new rather than misheard. Parents and the school team can work together to determine how to best assist the child with ongoing vocabulary growth.

4. Having optimally fit hearing aids or speech processor maps will provide the child with as complete a speech signal as possible. Audiological evaluation at least annually and whenever the child's hearing ability seems to have possibly changed is vital as the hearing loss can (and often does) change over time.

5. Children have a wide variety of abilities to attend to instruction throughout the day. Teachers need to be aware that the child with hearing loss will experience

varying levels of attention and distractibility that are not related to an attention deficit disorder (ADD or ADHD) in most cases. Attention issues are an outgrowth of fatigue from the need to continuously put more effort into listening to hear in addition to the effort to comprehend what is heard. Children with hearing loss have two listening jobs—not just one! How much effort the child must put into listening to hear will depend on his or her hearing loss, language ability, and of course, the classroom listening environment.

Addressing Challenges in the Learning Environment

All professionals who have the responsibility to educate children with hearing loss should recognize that children with hearing loss have challenges in the learning environment that are barriers to their equal access to instruction and academic success. As has been mentioned, all children in the classroom have the challenge of listening in order to comprehend information presented verbally while in the presence of inappropriate levels of background noise or reverberation. Listening is a primary gateway to learning and although we cannot expect the millions of classrooms across the country to provide ideal acoustic conditions, we can acknowledge that inadequate classroom acoustics provide a clearly identifiable learning barrier. Educational environments that have inadequate acoustic conditions can cause irreparable erosion of achievement for children with hearing loss by preventing them from optimally accessing verbal instruction. The ability to achieve in the classroom is related directly to the ability to access verbal instruction. Therefore, classroom acoustics is a vital consideration when determining the need for accommodations and specialized instruction that a student with hearing loss will need for success. (Refer to Figure 4-5 for an illustration of a student listening with the challenges of distance and noise.)

Distance and Background Noise

In order to achieve a +15 S/N the loudness of the signal and/or the loudness of the noise must be controlled to allow verbal instruction to be perceived consistently at this acceptable listening level. It is a fact that the loudness of a sound decreases at the ear level of the listener as the listener moves farther away from the source. The voice of a person who is close to the listener will be heard more loudly than the voice of a person who is farther away. The child with hearing loss needs verbal instruction to be delivered as close to the ears as possible if that spoken information is to be perceived without degradation due to distance. How close is close enough? As was seen in Figure 4-5, in a typical classroom the teacher's mouth would have to be 12" from a listener's ears for a +15 dB S/N to be achieved and as close as 4.5" for +24 dB S/N to occur, assuming that the ambient noise level was a typical SPL of 60 dB.

The 2002 National Standard for classroom acoustics specifies that the background noise level in an unoccupied classroom is not to exceed 35 dB, which is substantially lower than the background level of 60 dB. The closer the ambient noise level is to 35 dB the easier it is for students to hear one another and the teacher. Also, in this day and age of cooperative learning and group projects, it's important for children to hear not only the teacher, but also their peers.

Controlling noise is only part of the problem. Remember that the prolonged sound reflections caused by excessive reverberation will also add noise to an active classroom and can interfere with understanding the speech of classmates and the teacher. With an appropriate reverberation time and level of background noise, it's possible for talkers to be farther away than 12" and for the children to still perceive speech at a +15 dB S/N. Therefore, it's critical that background noise, reverberation time and distance be addressed for the listener with hearing loss. Figure 4-7 illustrates a classroom bubble without use of S/N enhancing technology.

Figure 4-7: Representation of a child listening with the challenges of distance from the teacher and classroom noise and reverberation (student's listening bubble).

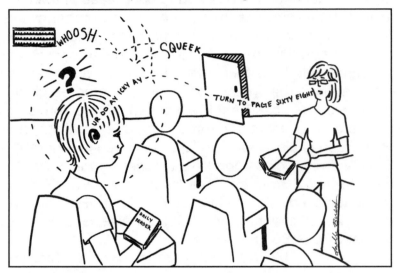

S/N Enhancing Technology

The most effective way to provide the necessary S/N for all students in a classroom is to reduce the unoccupied ambient noise level to 35 dB or less. For the child with hearing loss an additional way to address S/N ratio is to place a microphone close to the teacher's mouth and transmit her voice by FM radio waves as though her mouth is really close to the child's ears. This is accomplished with personal S/N enhancing devices. Personal FM devices continue to evolve much like other miniaturized electronics resulting in at least several companies manufacturing a variety of styles of FM systems. To locate information on different manufacturers, a web browser search is suggested using the following key words: FM system manufacturer educational hearing impaired.

The Federal Communications Commission has defined a band of radio frequencies just for use by devices used by people with hearing loss so, even though the devices use a radio signal, there isn't competition from regular radio or most other devices that use FM signals (e.g., baby monitors, garage door openers). In general, FM devices have two parts: the microphone transmitter worn by the teacher that transmits her voice across distance, and the receiver worn by the child or placed close to the child. The receiver of the personal FM device delivers the teacher's speech signal either directly to the child's hearing aids or the cochlear implant speech processor or it can also deliver the teacher's speech signal from a small speaker (like a computer speaker) that sits on the child's desk. The school district's educational audiologist or the child's clinical audiologist can provide more information about the variety of FM systems that are available and may be appropriate for the child to try in a classroom setting. FM systems are typically used during a trial period for 2-4 weeks and information is gathered from the child and/or teacher on how beneficial the device is to the child in the classroom at the end of the trial period. At this time there's not one type of FM system that works best for all children and their educational situations, so it's important to consider the options with an open mind and to allow the child and school staff to experiment until a truly beneficial arrangement can be determined.

In general, when a student with hearing loss uses a personal FM device, it does not benefit the rest of the children in the classroom. Even for persons with hearing loss, listening in a noisy classroom (background noise above 35 dB) while using FM technology will still cause problems. This technology does not "fix" the issues of background noise and reverberation and cannot be considered a substitute that will address all of the listening needs of the child with hearing loss, especially if reverberation greater than 0.6 seconds is present.

There are different types of S/N enhancing devices that deliver the teacher's voice to the student with hearing loss and it is important to recognize that distance is a key factor when considering the merits of these devices. A device that delivers the amplified teacher's voice from loudspeakers near the ceiling (a classroom sound field FM or infrared device) will still be requiring the student with hearing loss to perceive that amplified signal across the distance from the loudspeaker to the child's personal amplification. This distance will almost always be beyond the critical distance for listening. Even a S/N enhancing device that delivers sound from a small speaker on the student's desk still requires the student with hearing loss to perceive that signal across the distance from the desktop to his or her hearing aids or cochlear implant(s), but importantly, a desktop signal is likely to be within the critical listening distance in the classroom. In addition to achieving an ambient noise level of 35 dB, the only S/N enhancing technique that doesn't require listening over distance as a factor is the type that presents the teacher's voice directly by direct input to the child's hearing aids or cochlear implant(s).

Addressing Distance, Noise and Reverberation

There are three acoustic issues that occur in the classroom that can pose a barrier to the listener with hearing loss thereby reducing speech perception:

- distance from the teacher;
- background noise; and
- reverberation

Means by which each of these issues can be addressed will follow.

Background Noise and Reverberation

Results from a study (Finitzo-Hieber and Tillman, 1978) illustrate how background noise and reverberation can affect the listening of children with normal hearing and those with hearing loss. Children in this study had a moderate degree of hearing loss (40-70 dB) and wore one hearing aid. Scores are in percent correct for children repeating words while listening in three levels of noise (0 dB S/N, +6 dB S/N, +12 dB S/N and quiet) in settings that had three different reverberation times (Quiet, 0.4 seconds, 1.2 seconds). The quiet conditions were accomplished by the children repeating words in a sound booth, similar to what is done in a hearing evaluation. A reverberation time of 0.6 seconds for a classroom less than 10,000 cubic feet and an unoccupied noise level of 35 dB to achieve a +15 dB S/N level are the requirements specified in the 2002 National Standard for classroom acoustics. Although +12 S/N is less than the recommended S/N ratio of 15 dB, it is achievable in most classrooms that have periods of quiet in which the teacher's voice is 12 dB louder than the generated background noise, for example, by the ventilation system.

The average scores for children with normal hearing and with hearing loss under these different listening conditions are included in Appendix 4-A. As can be seen by the results shown in Appendix 4-B represented by bar graphs, even in a situation in which reverberation time was considered to be good (0.4 seconds), children had speech recognition scores that were substantially lower than what would be necessary for a child who needs to listen competitively within a classroom setting. The level of reverberation and noise really does result in a difference in listening accuracy!

Thus, it's important for parents and teachers of children with hearing loss to be aware of how adequate the classroom reverberation time and typical noise level is for the child with hearing loss. Compromising on reverberation time and/or on background noise will compromise the amount of instruction that is heard and learning that takes place.

The challenge of listening in excessive reverberation and noise continues to be present today, even with modern hearing aids and cochlear implants that provide substantial improvements in listening benefit over the analog hearing aid that these students wore in just one ear when the research was performed in 1978.

A recent study (Anderson, Goldstein, Colodzin, Iglehart, 2005) was conducted with children who wore modern hearing aids or cochlear implants and were successful students educated in the regular classroom without need for specialized instruction. Results are summarized in Appendix 4-C. The children had hearing losses ranging from mild through profound. They were asked to repeat 5-word sentences when either their hearing aids or their cochlear implant while in the presence of constant background noise at +6 S/N or +10 S/N and at 0.4 RT and 1.1 RT. This study was different from the 1978 study in that each child was not tested in classroom spaces with different reverberation times. There were different groups of students participating in each of these three experiments. Because of this the effects of reverberation are not very evident— only if each child was tested in each of these environments would the effects of differing reverberation times be seen.

Within the population of children with hearing loss, speech perception accuracy varies widely from individual to individual due to a variety of factors including degree of hearing loss, experience with listening, and motivation to really listen. Such a wide range in performance can be seen in the results of this study included as Appendix 4-C. Take time to consider the wide variety of hearing losses and how successfully each child performed. If you're aware of the word discrimination ability of a child when he or she is tested in a sound booth under +10 S/N conditions, then consider the child's potential performance compared to other children in this study. Speech perception ability as reflected in the percent of words repeated correctly when listening to sentences by the 22 children with hearing aids ranged from 46% to 98% and the speech perception of the 6 children with cochlear implants ranged from 46% to 95%. What is the speech perception ability in quiet of the child that you are concerned about? The overall speech perception score averaged 83% correct with personal devices with 2/3 of these very successful students with modern sensory devices missing 10% to 30% of the speech presented when using only their personal device.

What percentage of speech does a child really need to perceive and still learn competitively with classroom peers? This is a valid question for children with normal hearing who are learning in very noisy classrooms as well as those with hearing loss who are learning in even minimally noisy and reverberant settings. We can predict that children who perceive less of the teacher's voice and therefore less verbal instruction will need to expend extra effort on listening and trying to understand the instruction or they'll suffer increasing learning gaps. We can also predict that any child who has language, attention or additional learning challenges that require them to already expend more effort to comprehend verbal instruction will be at an even greater disadvantage in a setting where effort must be expended to hear and comprehend.

In times past it was all but assumed that children with hearing loss would require self-contained instruction due to their substantial language delays or would need to have visual communication methods because enough of the auditory signal could not be accessed for them to competitively learn with their peers. With early identification of hearing loss, early amplification and early intervention services, this scenario no longer needs to become a reality for children with hearing loss. The "No Child Left Behind Act" of 2002 requires schools to make genuine progress in closing the persistent achievement gap between students who are disadvantaged (or disabled) and their peers. Thus, school districts working in combination with informed proactive parents will be more likely than ever before to be motivated to identify gaps in learning and address them effectively. They may also be more willing to be proactive to prevent the predictable erosion in the achievement of children with hearing loss because access to verbal instruction is compromised.

The results of the 1978 study previously mentioned showed that the children with normal hearing in a setting with +12 S/N and 0.4 RT perceived on average about 83% of verbal instruction. Logically, in order to receive equal access to verbal instruction and not experience erosion in language and academic skills over time, the child with hearing loss should also perceive 83% of verbal instruction or more. This 83% average listening score was what was found in the 2005 study by the 22 students using only their hearing aids or cochlear implants. In actuality, the percent of word recognition a child with hearing loss is able to achieve in a quiet (sound booth) setting is his or her optimal listening ability. The child with normal hearing can be expected to achieve 95+% on word recognition tests conducted in a sound booth. The difference between a child's optimal listening ability in the quiet of a sound booth and the presumed almost 100% word recognition abilities of their classmates represents the extra challenge posed by the child's hearing loss. Equal access to verbal instruction lay in trying to present speech with the optimal clarity possible to the child with hearing loss.

Perceiving speech with optimal recognition will typically be needed to accommodate the reduction in intensity and clarity of speech caused by the hearing loss in order to prevent erosion in achievement over time. Instead, too often, students with hearing loss "make do" with speech perception that's 10%, 20% or 30+% poorer than their class peers and then must also deal with speech perception that's further diminished by poor acoustic conditions in the classroom. As will be discussed next in Chapter 5, schools have a responsibility to provide all students with equal access to instruction. For the student with hearing impairment, this means finding ways to restore this "lost percentage of verbal instruction."

The study reported in 2005 (Anderson, Goldstein, Colodzin, and Iglehart) investigated children's speech perception when using three different S/N enhancing devices (classroom soundfield, desktop FM and personal FM) to determine which device provided the most benefit to the students with hearing loss, thereby preventing lost percentage of verbal instruction (see Figures 4-8 and 4-9).

Each student was required to repeat 5-word sentences while listening to the three different S/N enhancing devices. In general, students performed best when the teacher's voice was presented within the critical listening distance (desktop FM or personal FM), and using a personal device alone or in combination with classroom soundfield amplification did not provide the benefit needed. Results of this study are shown in Appendix 4-D.

Hearing aids or cochlear implants alone, even those with recent technological advances, do not overcome the interfering effects of background noise and reverberation on speech perception of most children in classrooms. Children who perform very successfully in the regular classroom will still have a wide range of speech perception abilities. In the 2005 study children's average speech perception improved by 8% for desktop FM and 10% for personal FM. Although there was an 8% and 10% average, the range in improvement was from 0% to 36%—the degree of benefit can vary widely! The average performance of the six children with cochlear implants indicated poorer listening

Figure 4-8: Representation of a child listening with to the teacher's speech through a desk top FM system (student's listening bubble with desk top FM).

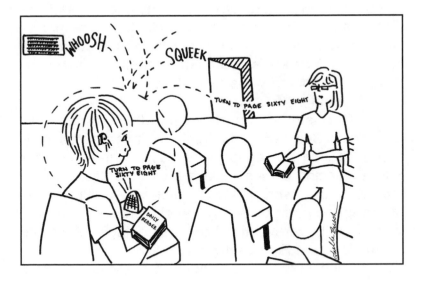

Figure 4-9: Representation of a child listening with to the teacher's speech through a personal FM system (student's listening bubble with a personal FM).

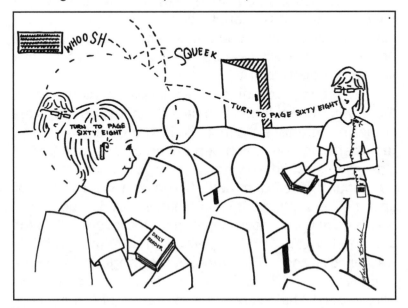

ability using classroom soundfield amplification over implant use alone. Average performance of the 22 children with hearing aids using classroom sound-field amplification indicated improvement within 2% of performance with hearing aids alone when class-room soundfield amplification is used. This was an insignificant improvement over use of personal hearing aids alone. Therefore, even though class-room sound field amplification improves the S/N in a classroom, this signal is delivered beyond the criti-cal distance for listening, thus allowing more inter-ference from the effects of reverberation.

Few parents would question that a gain of an average of 10% in speech perception is worth the extra effort to obtain and maintain use of a personal S/N enhancing device. Therefore, it is rarely, if ever, the responsible choice to deny the child with hear-ing loss this boost in speech perception. The dollar investment in equipment is justified by the necessi-ty to provide equal access to education for children with hearing loss. The individual's inherent skill at listening to speech in the presence of noise and reverberation and also the degree of effort that each student must expend to continuously "fill in the blanks," needs to be taken into consideration as decisions about S/N enhancing devices are made. When a listener is denied the maximum amount of auditory information possible (an additional unknown percent of assistance could have been provided through the use of S/N enhancing technol-ogy) they're being denied equal access to verbal instruction. For children with hearing loss who learn through their ears like their classmates, being able to hear as much as possible of what their teachers and classmates say in the classroom is what allows them to be successful without increasing amounts of pull-out or other specialized instruction.

Reverberation

The problem of excessive reverberation time cannot be solved through simply buying the "best" hearing aids, speech processor or S/N enhancing technology. Excessive reverberation smears the speech signal that reaches these devices and they cannot "unsmear" it. Decreasing background noise in a classroom will not make the room quiet if there are excessive reflective surfaces that prolong the sound. Only increasing the amount of sound-absorbing surfaces will help. Children are much more susceptible to the smearing effect than are adults, and children with hearing loss are the most vulnerable of all. The greater the distance between the microphone on the child's personal device and the teachers lips, the greater the effect that excessive RT will have on speech signal clarity. Children with hearing loss should be educated in classrooms with 0.6 seconds or less of reverberation time. There has been some evidence that reverberation times of 0.3 to 0.4 seconds are ideal for children with hearing loss, although this RT is usually unrealistic in school settings. Therefore, in a classroom with reverberation exceeding 0.6 seconds, it would be most effective to:

1. Increase the absorptive surfaces in the room (i.e., add acoustic wall panels, carpeting, better ceiling tile, etc.) to reduce the reverberation to 0.6 seconds or less.

2. Reduce background noise (to a level of 35 dB or less when unoccupied if possible) in the classroom. For children with hearing loss educated in a classroom with reverberation time greater than 0.6 seconds, placement of the microphone of the S/N enhancing technology is critical (but will not fix the RT problem).

3. Consider employing a microphone placed close to the teacher's mouth (called a boom microphone) rather than a lapel microphone and a S/N enhancement device placed as close as possible to the child's ear (e.g. a personal FM receiver).

S/N-enhancing technology cannot solve the acoustic smearing or noise caused in a classroom by excessive reverberation that results in barriers to equal access to verbal instruction. All three of these steps will help address the ability of students to perceive and comprehend the teacher's speech, but use of a boom microphone by only the teacher will not address what is said by classmates or anyone in the class who's not currently using the microphone of the S/N enhancing device. A smaller classroom with fewer students may provide an easy acoustic solution to allow the child with hearing loss to hear classmates' voices. However, this may not be the least restrictive educational setting for the student.

The S/N-enhancing device cannot bridge the distance for listening during cooperative learning activities, class discussions and even hearing social commentary and conversation. Pass-around microphones are very effective when used, but often slow the dynamic of active discussion to the point where the classmates, teacher and child become frustrated and the child with hearing loss can become embarrassed. Too often pass-around microphones fall into disuse over time, especially during times when children are talking to one another. If a child relies primarily on listening for learning and communication, then reducing background noise and controlling reverberation time in the classroom are necessary for him or her to access as much of this active social and cooperative learning communication as possible.

The amount of reverberation can only be controlled by reducing the amount of reflective surface area that's present in the classroom. It's recommended that an acoustical engineer be consulted about how best to achieve an acceptable reverberation time (0.6 seconds RT or less) in individual school situations. In general, for typical classrooms with 8 to 12 foot ceilings, the surface area of the acoustic treatment (ceilings, floor, wall surfaces) should be about 80% to

120% of the surface area of the floor. The presence of good quality acoustic tile on the ceiling is the single most effective means by which this can be achieved. If acoustically treating the ceiling does not sufficiently reduce RT, then single acoustic panels can be installed on the upper portions of two or more walls until up to 120% portion of the surface area is achieved. [For more information on the amount of acoustical treatment to apply to a classroom to achieve the required maximum reverberation time of 0.6 seconds for a typical classroom refer to Annex C of the 2002 National Standard at *http://www.access-board.gov/acoustic*, and/or you may consult with an acoustical engineer.]

When reverberation was first described in this chapter the benefits of having some reflection of sound was mentioned. In lecture-style classrooms in the upper grades where the teacher is stationary and there are no cooperative learning activities, most of the ceiling surface should be covered with good acoustic tile, but it could also include a hard-surfaced panel to reflect the teacher's voice to the rear portion of the classroom. The reflective panel would also be slightly sloped to further direct the teacher's voice and would be made of a hard material such as plasterboard or plywood. Sound-absorbing material (such as acoustic tile) would surround the reflective panel.

For an active classroom where the teacher roams among the students and there are many group activities, other means to control excessive background noise are needed. Carpeting in the classroom and medium quality acoustic tile can control reverberation and also reduce the generation of background noise due to foot and desk movement. Sometimes just by putting 3"- 4" blocks under the bottom of the white boards or chalkboards on the walls of the classrooms will help because the angle of this reflective surface will cause sound to be reflected to the ceiling and absorbed by the acoustic tile more directly and can thereby reduce how long sound is prolonged in a classroom.

Schools that don't want to install carpeting in class-rooms can achieve control of excessive reverberation by:

1. installation of high quality acoustic ceiling tile;
2. placement of additional absorbent wall panels on the upper portion of walls; and
3. by putting tennis balls or a similar solution (e.g., "QuietFeet"™ *http//www.acousticresources.net*) on each leg of student chairs and desks to reduce the amount of noise generated in the classroom.

It's much less expensive to build schools with appropriate acoustic treatment and noise control than it is to retrofit many single classrooms or remodel whole schools. Remodeling schools to improve acoustics is expensive primarily because the ventilation systems purchased through 'value engineering' are typically the biggest culprits in producing unacceptable levels of background noise. Most often there's a lack of consideration of the need for quality absorptive surfaces which results in the purchase of cheap acoustic tile, or worse yet, building open-plan schools.

Schools with open plan classroom designs will have excessive reverberation and interference from noise because of the lack of walls to block transmission of sound from space to space. Although children with hearing loss in these schools may have the skills and speech perception ability to succeed in the mainstream, the acoustic environment is a barrier that cannot be overcome adequately through seating and technology. Open plan settings are inappropriate for the education of students with hearing loss or other problems affecting auditory speech processing. With increasing numbers of children with hearing loss being educated in their home schools, it's appropriate for adequate acoustic treatment to be considered for all new and remodeled school building projects. It makes sense to build schools in which students can clearly hear their teachers.

All children deserve to be able to hear their teachers clearly. Although classroom soundfield amplification will improve the S/N for all students, it is not the answer to improving inappropriate acoustics due to excessive reverberation or high levels of background noise. To use an analogy, think of a classroom that has no windows and is only lit by a 40-watt light bulb. Students can see the teacher, but cannot distinguish all her expressions and movements easily, clearly or effortlessly. If you put glasses on all of the students so that it's easier for them to see the teacher, it would help a bit, but wouldn't address the real problem of poor lighting. If you provide the teacher with a flashlight, this would ease some situations, but again would not address the real problem of having inadequate light to illuminate to a level necessary to see and distinguish detail with ease. In a similar manner, although classroom soundfield amplification helps students with normal hearing to hear their teacher, it doesn't address the real problem of poor acoustics. Children with normal hearing in classrooms that have 0.6 RT and background noise up to 45 dB (10 dB more than the 35 dB allowable noise standard) may experience marked benefit in easier listening through the excessive background noise. However, greater RT or background noise levels won't be solved by classroom soundfield amplification. Indeed, introducing an additional sound source in a classroom with excessive reverberation will exacerbate the listening challenges rather than solve them. For most children with hearing loss, classroom soundfield amplification doesn't provide enough S/N improvement to meet their needs and continues to allow degradation of the speech signal due to listening over distance.

Individualized Assessment of Listening Difficulty in Typical Situations

Education in the 21st century requires mastery in perceiving and processing massive quantities of information that's then integrated into previous knowledge and applied through the use of critical thinking skills. Listening is the primary gateway through which most children learn. The acoustic environment can, and does, pose a barrier to children performing their best in school. As can be seen in Appendix 4-C, speech perception abilities of children with hearing loss vary widely and therefore need to be considered individually. This can be achieved in a few ways.

As a part of a child's hearing evaluation the audiologist can have the child repeat words or short sentences in the sound booth under different listening conditions and then compare the percent correct. These conditions could be:

1. in quiet;
2. +5 S/N (typical poor acoustics);
3. +10 S/N (typical fair acoustics);
4. +15 S/N (appropriate acoustics); and
5. +20 S/N (simulated listening with a personal S/N enhancing device).

The changes in the word recognition in percent can be very useful for parents and school teams to consider in regard to the child's acoustic setting and S/N enhancement device needs.

Word or sentence recognition under different listening conditions can also be obtained informally, and in some ways more functionally, by an educational audiologist, speech language pathologist or teacher of the deaf or hard-of-hearing. This Functional Listening Evaluation is performed by having the child repeat words or phrases at different distances and levels of background noise, when the child is watching the words as they're verbally presented and when the child is not allowed to speechread. The procedure is described in the assessment section of *http://www.colorado.edu/slhs/mdnc/.*

Parents and school professionals can also use observation and interview techniques to gauge the degree to which the child with hearing loss can function in typically noisy situations. At the time of this writing, there are several tests that can be downloaded at no cost from *http://www.hear2learn.com.*

Parents of children age 4 months to 3 years can use the Early Listening Function (ELF) instrument as a means to systematically observe how the "listening bubble" of their child changes as they detect different sounds in quiet and in the presence of noise. This early awareness of the child's ability to detect sound in noisy situations can be very valuable as a means for parents to describe the effect of the child's hearing loss on listening and learning, especially as the child enters community child care or preschool settings.

Parents of children age 3 years through elementary school can use the Children's Home Inventory of Listening Difficulties (CHILD) as a means to identify the degree of difficulty their child appears to have when perceiving and processing speech in typical home situations. Older children (i.e., age 8+) can also rate their own listening ability in situations described in the CHILD test. Comparing the responses of parents and children can provide insights into self-esteem, awareness of level of listening difficulty, and effects of hearing loss on peer relationships. The information gathered on the CHILD can assist parents in advocating for acoustic, technology, and accommodation needs as these children enter school and in planning for their needs in preschool, kindergarten or early elementary school classrooms.

Finally, the Listening Inventory For Education (LIFE) has two forms; a Student Appraisal and a Teacher Appraisal. The LIFE Student Appraisal is administered via interview of the child by a school professional. The child is asked questions about how well he or she can hear and understand in different listening situations typically occurring at school. Most children starting at about 8 years old are able to rate themselves on this type of survey, although the value of the information is only as valid as the child is honest when answering the questions. Questions relate to quiet and noisy situations during verbal instruction and in nonacademic situations. On the second page (or reverse side) of the Student Appraisal there are recommended self-advocacy techniques that students can use when they encounter difficulties in these different situations. Responses on the LIFE can be useful as a basis for individualized accommodations needed in daily classroom listening situations. The LIFE Teacher Appraisal is a post-test form to be used as a means of determining degree of benefit when new or newly adjusted personal sensory devices or S/N-enhancement devices are being tried. After trying the new device or a newly adjusted device for a few weeks, the teacher completes the LIFE Teacher Appraisal. On this form the teacher indicates if he or she has observed changes in the child's behavior during different classroom listening situations. The responses to the LIFE teacher and student appraisal forms can be used in combination with functional listening evaluation information as the parents and school team consider the degree to which the child is able to successfully access verbal instruction and the need for accommodations and technology to support optimal access.

Parents who are aware of their child's strengths and limitations as the child functions in typical listening, learning and social environments can be powerful advocates when working with the schools, just as teachers with this awareness can be truly effective as they consider the individual needs of the child with hearing loss. The challenges faced by learners with hearing loss are great, but teams of parents and educators can collaborate successfully to help make each child's future bright. Parents can fully participate in planning an educational program and learning environment best suited for an appropriate public education in which the child will have equal access to verbal instruction. In the 21st century, the possibilities for school success need not be limited for the child with hearing loss!

References

American National Standards Institute (2002). S12.60 – 2002, <u>Acoustical performance criteria, design requirements, and guidelines for schools</u>.

Anderson, K. L., Goldstein, H., Colodzin, L., & Iglehart, F. (2005). Benefit of S/N enhancing devices to speech perception of children listening in a typical classroom with hearing aids or a cochlear implant. <u>Journal of Educational Audiology</u> (12), 14-28.

Crandell, C., & Smaldino, J. (1995). Speech perception in the classroom. In C. Crandell, J. Smaldino, C. Flexer (Ed.), *Sound-Field FM Amplification: Theory and Practical Applications* (pp 29-48). San Diego, CA: Singular.

Finitzo-Hieber, T., & Tillman, T. (1978). Room acoustics effects on monosyllabic word discrimination ability for normal and hearing-impaired children. <u>Journal of Speech and Hearing Research</u>, 21, 440-458.

Nabelek, A. and Nabelek, I. (1985). Room acoustics and speech perception. In J. Katz (Ed.), *Handbook of Clinical Audiology* (3rd Edition). Baltimore, MD: Williams and Wilkins.

Appendix 4-A

Word recognition scores for single words expressed in percent correct for children with normal hearing and for children with moderate hearing loss listening at different levels of reverberation and S/N.

Test Condition	Normal Hearing	Hearing Loss
RT = 0.0 Seconds (hearing test booth)		
Quiet	94.5	83.0
+12 S/N	89.2	70.0
+6 S/N	79.7	59.5
0 S/N	60.2	39.0
RT = 0.4 Second (appropriate RT)		
Quiet	92.5	74.0
+12 S/N	82.8	60.2
+6 S/N	71.3	52.2
0 S/N	47.4	27.8
RT = 1.2 Second (too reverberant)		
Quiet	76.5	45.0
+12 S/N	68.8	41.2
+6 S/N	54.2	27.0
0 S/N	29.7	11.2

Source: Table adapted from Finitzo-Hieber and Tillman (1978).

Appendix 4-B

Results of study using three reverberation times and four noise levels (Finitzo-Hieber and Tillman, 1978).

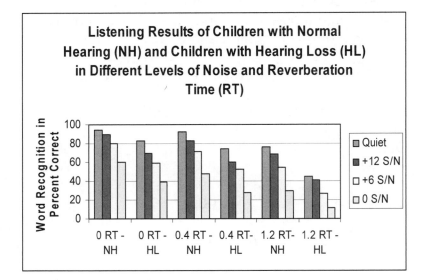

Listening Results of Children with Normal Hearing (NH) and Children with Hearing Loss (HL) in Different Levels of Noise and Reverberation Time (RT)

Appendix 4-C

Word recognition scores in sentences expressed in percent correct for children with hearing loss wearing hearing aids or a cochlear implant when listening at different levels of reverberation and S/N with personal amplification devices alone or each of three S/N enhancing devices.

Partici-pant #	Pers. Device	Pers. Dev Only	Classrm SF	Desktop FM	Pers. FM
+6 S/N 1.1 RT					
1	HA	95.7	95.7	92.0	92.4
2	HA	89.0	88.3	97.0	99.3
3	HA	82.7	79.3	87.0	88.3
4	HA	98.0	96.3	97.7	98.0

(Continued next page)

Appendix 4-C (con't)

Partici-pant #	Pers. Device	Pers. Dev Only	Classrm SF	Desktop FM	Pers. FM
5	HA	90.3	91.0	94.7	92.0
6	HA	72.7	75.7	85.0	81.0
7	HA	92.7	92.0	94.0	96.0
8	HA	73.2	88.3	94.7	92.3
9	HA	91.0	85.0	89.3	94.3
mean	HA	87.3	88.0	92.4	92.6

+10 S/N   1.1 RT

10	HA	68.0	74.6	84.0	86.7
11	HA	76.0	71.3	86.7	95.3
12	HA	80.6	82.0	92.0	95.3
13	HA	89.3	84.0	92.7	96.7
14	HA	93.3	95.3	98.7	100.0
15	HA	88.7	82.0	97.3	89.3
16	HA	90.7	93.3	99.3	97.3
17	HA	72.7	82.0	97.3	94.7
mean	HA	82.4	83.1	93.5	94.4

+10 S/N   0.4 RT

18	CI	72.0	74.2	94.0	92.0
19	CI	86.0	72.0	90.0	84.0
20	HA	96.0	82.0	92.0	100.0
21	CI	95.0	84.0	100.0	100.0
22	CI	79.9	30.0	60.0	76.0
23	HA	46.0	50.0	78.0	82.0
24	HA	68.0	92.0	86.0	100.0
25	CI	46.0	62.0	84.0	100.0
26	HA	90.0	80.0	96.0	92.0
27	CI	86.0	68.0	96.0	92.0
28	HA	90.0	76.0	88.0	92.0
Mean	combined	77.7	70.0	87.6	91.8
Mean	HA only	78.0	76.0	88.0	93.2
Mean	CI only	77.5	65.0	87.3	90.7
Total Mean (Standard Deviation)		82.13 (13.55)	79.51 (14.46)	90.83 (8.18)	92.82 (6.33)

Appendix 4-D

Results of 2005 study of 28 children with mild to profound hearing loss using hearing aids or cochlear
implants and 3 different S/N enhancing devices.

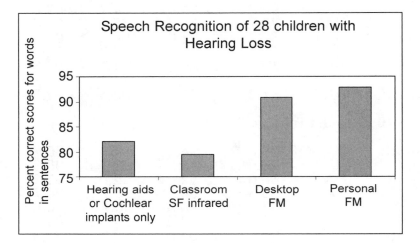

Chapter 5
What Parents Should Know:

The Educational System[*]

Cheryl DeConde Johnson, Ed. D.

Dr. Johnson is currently a supervisor and consultant with the Colorado Department of Education where her responsibilities include services to students with hearing disabilities. She provides technical assistance and leadership for hearing loss education, educational interpreting, and educational audiology services statewide. Prior to employment at the Department of Education, she worked for 22 years as an educational audiologist and hearing consultant in the Greeley-Evans School District 6 in Greeley, Colorado as well as a Colorado Hearing Resource Coordinator (CO-Hear) and parent facilitator for the Colorado Home Intervention Program (CHIP) for D/HH.

Dr. Johnson's special interests include childhood auditory function and its associated implications, management of children with hearing loss in education settings, and accountability in hearing loss education. She is a co-author of the Educational Audiology Handbook, as well as numerous other articles and chapters. She consults and frequently presents nationally and internationally on topics related to reform of education for children with hearing loss and educational audiology. Dr. Johnson also maintains adjunct faculty appointments with the University of Colorado and Central Michigan University. Her inspiration and work continues to be influenced by her daughter who was born with hearing loss as a result of Rubella.

[*]Information contained in this chapter is intended to provide guidance and should not be construed as anything more. Attorneys who specialize in special education case law should be consulted in legal matters that pertain to specific situations.

- Parents are a child's best advocate.
- Parents need information to make informed decisions for their child.
- A good education program considers the parents as equal partners.
- Behind most successful children are parents who value education.
- A strong parent/professional partnership sets the stage for a positive educational experience.

If one believes the statements above, then it's easy to recognize how important the parent's role will be throughout a child's education. However, navigating the legal aspects of early intervention and educational systems can often be confusing. To add to the confusion, legal interpretations may vary from state to state, county to county, and school district to school district resulting in regulations that often seem inconsistent. Transition periods, e.g., between the early intervention system for infants and toddlers, and the school-age system, and from high school to adult life further add to the complexity of systems and services.

Key Concepts in Educational Services and Programming

IDEA

It is important to identify and understand some key laws and concepts that are essential to our understanding of the education of children with hearing loss. The Individuals with Disabilities Education Act (IDEA) is the landmark legislation that defines the procedural aspects pertaining to the identification, assessment and provision of services to children with hearing loss. This law is divided into two parts, Part B which pertains to children and youth age 3 to 21, and Part C for infants and toddlers, birth to age 3. There are many similarities between the two sections. However, an important distinction is that Part C is focused on services that families need to support their child and Part B is more child-centered addressing how the school program will provide the services and supports that are needed. IDEA also provides important protections to families with regard to the education of children with hearing loss. Once eligibility has been established, the Individual Family Service Plan (IFSP) for infants and toddlers, and the Individual Educational Program (IEP) for children and youth 3 to age 21, are the legal documents that specify the services and supports that are provided.

The IFSP is developed by the parents in conjunction with the professionals that are involved with the child. A service coordinator is assigned to coordinate the IFSP and to assist the family in identifying and accessing services. The IFSP is reviewed every six months and rewritten annually. It includes the following basic components:

- *Present Levels of Development*—describes what the child does well and things that are difficult within the areas of motor, speech and language, cognition, social-emotional and self-help skills.
- *Concerns and Priorities*—based on the family's concerns, with input from the professionals involved with the family such as the child's audiologist and the early intervention provider, immediate priorities are identified. It is paramount that the early intervention provider be knowledgeable and experienced in early intervention with children with hearing loss.
- *Expected Outcomes*—an action plan that addresses each priority, including an outcome statement and strategies for how it will be

achieved within the child and family's everyday routines, activities and places.

- *Supports and Services*—identifies the early intervention service provider/program, including audiology, the activity provided, how the services are delivered, the frequency (such as once/week) and duration (length of each session), start and end dates, and the funding source. The IFSP also include the steps necessary to support the transition of the child to preschool or other appropriate services.

The IEP (for children 3-21 years) is developed by the team of school professionals that will work with the child along with the parents. It is reviewed annually, rewritten every three years, and includes the following components:

- *Present Level of Educational Performance*—a description of current educational status which includes cognitive skills, linguistic ability, emotional behavior, social skills, behavior and physical ability. The description may include both informal (anecdotal information such as observations and questionnaires) as well as formal information (testing data, grades).
- *Annual Measurable Goals and Short-Term Objectives*—considered the backbone of the IEP as the goals determine the focus of the specialized instruction and the objectives describe the steps taken to achieve them. Objectives must be specific, measurable, attainable, employ methods that are known to be effective, and include a timetable of when they will be achieved.

Example: Goal—Susan will improve her reading skills.

Objective: Susan will gain 9 months by May 1 in her reading comprehension abilities using reading program X as measured by the program's pre-post reading comprehension assessment.

- *Special Education and Related Services*—identifies the actual services provided, which members of the team will be providing the services, the amount of time (such as once per day or once per week), and the duration of each session. Services include audiology, speech-language therapy and counseling, in addition to the instructional services provided by the teacher of the deaf/hard-of-hearing.
- *Instructional Setting or Placement and Extent to which the Child Participates in the General Education Class*—where will the special education services be provided? Placement can range from the child's home school to a center program for students with hearing loss to a special school. Within that placement, the services could be provided in the child's general education classroom if it's a regular school, in a specialized classroom in a regular or special school, or a combination of both.
- *Other Components on the IEP*—these include how parents will be regularly informed of their child's progress, how the child will participate in district and state assessments, and how assistive technology will be provided. In addition, for children with hearing loss, the IEP team must consider special communication needs (see section: Communication Considerations page 158 in this chapter).

No Child Left Behind

While IDEA provides procedural protections, it does not directly assure quality education programs. No Child Left Behind (NCLB) was passed by Congress to increase accountability of school districts for student achievement. These concepts are important because they impact all students regardless of whether they are in special education or not. Furthermore, most students with hearing loss receive the majority of their education in the general education classroom. Some of the most noteworthy provisions of NCLB and the implications for students with hearing loss include the following:

1. *Accountability for results:* all children, including those with hearing loss, are included in the accountability equation. Student progress and achievement is measured by standardized tests for every child. Data from the annual assessments must be reported in annual report cards on school performance and on statewide progress. The report cards provide the parents and community information about the quality of schools, the qualifications of teachers, and progress in key subject areas. Data must be analyzed according to race, gender, disabilities and other criteria to demonstrate progress that's being made to close the achievement gap between disadvantaged students and other student groups.

Implications for students with hearing loss:
- The accountability provision under NCLB has become a major factor toward improving achievement outcomes for students with hearing loss. For the first time, these students are being held to the same standard as their hearing peers. The implications are that these students must be taught using the same standards as hearing children and that they must have access

to the general education curriculum where these standards are taught. Access to the curriculum requires schools to provide the necessary supports that provide students with hearing loss accessibility. These include appropriate amplification and assistive technologies, acoustically and visually appropriate classrooms, qualified educational interpreters, note-taking services and other common accommodations utilized by students with hearing loss.

- Another implication of NCLB has been the analysis of performance data on statewide assessments. The requirement to look specifically at assessment data for students with hearing disabilities as compared to their hearing peers has clearly identified the gap in achievement between these groups. This process has forced schools to begin a critical analysis of practices used with children with hearing loss.

2. *Ensuring that every child can read.* The federal government's Reading First initiative is the basis for this provision. This initiative's foundation is the use of scientifically proven methods of reading instruction. Implications for students with hearing loss:

- While the Reading First initiative is based on scientifically proven methods, these methods may not be proven or appropriate for children with hearing loss. Several components of the reading program are auditory—based, clearly a disadvantage to some children with hearing loss.

3. *Strengthening teacher quality.* This part of NCLB requires teachers and other support staff in every public school classroom to be "highly qualified."

With shortages increasing in some special education areas, the reality of the provision makes it even more challenging. This law requires all special education teachers at the secondary level to have the content specialization in the areas where they are the student's primary subject matter teacher (e.g., math, English, social studies, science).

Implications for students with hearing loss:

- Students with hearing loss are benefiting from this highly qualified provision. The most impact is seen at the secondary content level described above and with the qualifications of educational interpreters. For content areas, teachers of the deaf/hard of hearing are now required to have teaching endorsements or special training in the content areas where they provide direct instruction. Since these provisions also affect related service providers, states are now implementing minimum standards for educational interpreters.

Communication Access:
The Most Essential Right for Children with Hearing Loss

Children are ultimately the focus of early intervention and educational programming. While early intervention programs include services and support for families, the emphasis remains on the child so that the goals of the parents (and later the child) can be realized. The disability of hearing loss often occurs when children are not provided access to communication and therefore fall behind in their development.

Communication access is the ability to connect and interact with people in one's environment. For children with hearing loss, the ability to connect and interact in a meaningful way requires some adaptations. The ability to access communication is necessary for the development of cognition, language and relationships with others. Every child with hearing loss has a basic human right to communication access (Siegel, 2002). As illustrated in Figure 5-1, communication access begins a process which can lead to either a path of development more like hearing children or to development that's delayed, requiring special supports. Communication access leads to language proficiency, cognitive development, social emotional well-being, academic competence and an opportunity to be a productive member of one's community. Alternatively, without communication access, development quickly breaks down. Children then require support from special education (IDEA) and as adults, from adult social and community services (vocational rehabilitation) to build these skills.

Figure 5-1: Communication Access as a Civil Rights Model.*

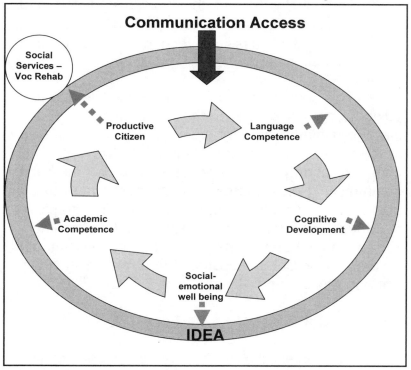

*Adapted from L. Siegel and C.D. Johnson, National Deaf Education Project, *www.ndepnow.org,* 2005.

Communication Considerations

IDEA regulations recognize the critical importance of communication access for children with hearing loss. Consideration of special factors [34CFR 300.324(a)(2)(iv)] requires the IEP team to consider the special communication needs of each child with hearing loss when developing the IEP. These considerations include:

- language and communication needs;
- opportunities for direct communications with peers and professional personnel in the child's language and communication mode;
- academic level
- full range of needs including opportunities for direct instruction in the child's language and communication mode; and
- the need for assistive technology devices and services.

This regulation is often the most relevant and powerful portion of the IEP for children with hearing loss. To achieve this right, parents must never waiver in their goal to assure that their child always has full communication access at home, in school, and in the community. Some states include a communication plan as part of their IEP and IFSP in order to assure that these considerations are addressed and the necessary adjustments in programming are made. [Examples of Communication Plans are included in Appendixes 5-A and 5-B.]

Parent's Rights

Fortunately, the role of parents has been continuously strengthened in IDEA. However, parents should never enter any stage of the special education process without being clear about their rights and protections under the laws. Through both Part C and Part B of the regulations, parents have the right to:

- examine all records pertaining to their child;
- receive prior written notice regarding the identification, evaluation, placement and provision of services;
- consent to initial evaluation and assessment and provision of services; and
- participate in all meetings involving eligibility and placement decisions.

In addition, parents in Part C have the right to decline services at any time. Parent permission requirements are summarized in Table 5-I.

Table 5-I. Activities that require and do not require parent permission.

Parent Permission Required	Parent Permission Not Required
• initial evaluation • initial placement • re-evaluation if in a program providing special education services (except that consent is not required if the school has taken reasonable measures to obtain parent consent and the parent fails to respond)	• reviewing existing data as part of an evaluation or re-evaluation • prior to giving a test or evaluation that is given to all students • continuation of special education services

Parents also have mediation and due process rights in any dispute regarding their child's IEP process with the school or early childhood agency. Mediation by a neutral person not employed by the school district may assist the parent and school in resolving differences regarding testing, placement or services. When a parent feels that a school district is violating procedures, they may file a complaint with their state department of education, Federal Complaints Officer. The written complaint process results in an independent binding decision to the school district and the parents.

School districts are required to provide parents a copy of their procedural safeguards upon the initial referral for evaluation, each notification of an IEP meeting, upon re-evaluation, and if a request for a due process hearing is made.

The Process at a Glance

Implementing services for a child with hearing loss is a multi-stage process. Figure 5-2 depicts the process for children ages 3-21 beginning with the referral process. Parents should seek additional clarification from their local school districts regarding how each of these steps is articulated in their community. It is important to be aware that children with hearing loss are not automatically eligible for services under IDEA. Eligibility must be demonstrated by identifying how the hearing loss adversely affects the child's ability to gain reasonable benefit from general education alone. For example, as a result of the hearing loss, the child must be delayed in academic content areas (reading, math, writing), language and communication or social/emotional areas. Each state develops its own specific eligibility criteria.

Children who have a hearing loss but do not demonstrate academic, language, communication or social problems to the extent that they meet eligibility requirements for special education, often qualify for Section 504 services under the Rehabilitation Act of 1973.

Figure 5-2. The IDEA and Section 504 placement process.*

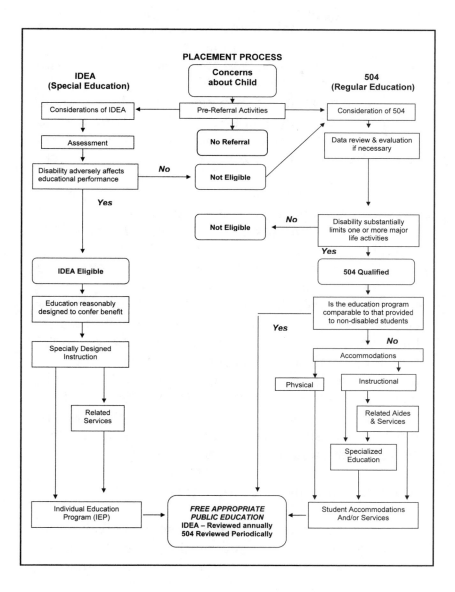

*From *Planning and Preparing Quality Individualized Education Programs*, Section I, p.6, 1996. Colorado Department of Education. Reprinted with permission.

These services are identified on a 504 Plan that explains the accommodations that will be provided so that the child can access his/her educational program (see accommodations and modifications discussion below for additional information). Services on a 504 Plan are provided through the general education program of the school; there is no special state or federal funding to support them.

One more important aspect of Part B for parents is parent counseling and training. This related service requires school districts to provide training and support to parents when it's necessary for their child to meet his/her IEP goals. Training in communication strategies, use of hearing aids or other assistive listening devices, sign language or cued speech are examples of services that parents might receive from their child's school.

The Part C system is more streamlined. Some infants and toddlers, including those with hearing loss, are automatically eligible for services based on their condition which is usually identified at or shortly after birth. Other infants and toddlers with developmental problems or disorders not present at birth go through an evaluation process to determine eligibility and subsequent development of the IFSP. The Part C authority varies from state to state but is usually the department of education, the department of health or other similar health and human service agency.

Accommodations and Modifications

These are terms used to describe how the general education program is altered to meet the individual needs of a student with disabilities. *Accommodations* refer to how the environment or instructional process will be adjusted so that the student can access learning. Common examples of accommodations for students with hearing loss include the use of FM systems, special seating in the classroom and other communication strategies to provide access to classroom instruction and discussion. Accommodations will be identified on the IEP or on a 504 plan for children who are not eligible for special education.

Modifications are ways the content is altered so that it's meaningful to students with disabilities. A modification for a student with hearing loss might be made for the phonics portion of a reading program to include more visual strategies or to utilize an alternative reading program. Additional accommodations and modifications are addressed in the IEP Checklist in Appendix 5-C.

Mainstreaming and Inclusion

Mainstreaming is a term that was prevalent in the seventies to mid-eighties to describe participation of students with disabilities in the general education classroom. In mainstreaming, children with hearing loss who required significant modifications to the general education curriculum received much of their instruction in a separate classroom where the content and delivery could be modified specifically for each child.

Inclusion evolved in the mid-eighties to focus on services in the general education classroom. In inclusion, the intent is to design the classroom and the specialized instruction to support the child. Table 5-II provides comparisons of *mainstreaming* and *inclusion* for further clarification between the two systems.

Co-teaching is a model that represents the best aspects of mainstreaming and inclusion. In co-teaching, a general education teacher and a deaf/hard of hearing teacher team together to teach all students in the classroom. The deaf/hard of hearing teacher brings the expertise to the classroom required for the students with hearing loss to assure that accommodations and modifications are applied appropriately and the general education teacher provides the expertise

Table 5-II: Comparison of *mainstreaming* and *inclusion*.

Mainstreaming	Inclusion
• Student's enrollment is under the teacher of students with hearing loss	• Student's enrollment is under the general education teacher
• Student's primary placement is the classroom for students with hearing loss	• Student's primary placement is the general education classroom; general education classroom is designed to support and accommodate the student
• Student attends general education classroom when he or she can benefit (often non-academic classes like PE, art)	• Student attends the special classroom for children with hearing loss only when instruction cannot be sufficiently provided within the general education classroom
• Student adapts to the general education program	• The general education program is designed to adapt to the student

for the subject content. In a well-functioning co-teaching classroom, it's difficult to identify who the students are who require special education due to the natural way in which these classrooms operate.

Teachers and parents must assure that children in the mainstream have sufficient language skills to benefit from instruction in the general classroom. A common guideline is acquired language skills within two years of the instructional level of the class. If the child's language skills are more than two years behind that of the classroom, it's unlikely that the teacher can sufficiently modify the instruction to provide the student a meaningful experience. Since the goal is academic integration it's critical that the children are prepared and supported to succeed in the general education classroom environment when determining placement. Because the philosophy of inclusion has often overridden these considerations, the US Department of Education published the Deaf Students Education Services Policy Guidance in 1992. This policy clarification was intended to clarify the education provisions of IDEA for children with hearing loss, including the determination of appropriate education for such children and the requirement that education be provided in the "least restrictive environment."

Least Restrictive Environment (LRE)

This basic tenet of IDEA requires that children be educated in the placement that most closely resembles that of their hearing peers, usually considered to be the general education classroom. However, given the language development concerns of children with hearing loss, the general education classroom may actually be more restrictive for children with hearing loss unless it is a communication accessible environment that provides meaningful opportunities for learning and participation. Therefore, educators of children with hearing loss have increasingly defined LRE as Language Rich Environment meaning that if the education setting isn't language rich (e.g., provides meaningful opportunities for learning and participation), it cannot be least restrictive. A comparison of poor and good language–rich environment examples is contained in Table 5-III.

Table 5-III. Poor and better language-rich environment examples.*

Thumbs Down

- Announcements given over a 20 year-old PA system.

- Oral deaf/hard of hearing students who don't need an interpreter and don't receive access support.

- Grouping students who have a hearing loss together to save money on interpreters and resources regardless of the individual need or mode of communication used by each student.

- Educational interpreters who do not meet minimum educational interpreter standards.

- No personal FM or only out-of-date "old style" auditory trainers used; school has cell phone antennae on the roof causing interference.

- High school students with hearing loss with no direct instruction due to lack of resources in rural areas.

- Administrative and finanancial considerations driving the IEP process and service delivery recommendations.

---

*Adapted from Hands & Voices, 2001. Reprinted with permission.

Thumbs Up

- Announcements through video came with signed interpretation, transmitted via a television in each classroom; real time captioning; written announcements delivered directly to students; teacher repeating the announcements.

- Real-time captioning and/or oral interpreter or "communication facilitator."

- Service delivery that is individualized and expectations that raise the bar for achievement to each student's highest potential.

- 100% of educational interpreters meet minimum standards.

- Digitally compatible, wireless FM systems available for every student who needs one; school district audiologist trained in current technology and has updated software to troubleshoot digital hearing aids.

- Honors-level science class taught in sign language via live satellite video.

- Decisions based on child's needs rather than what the existing program offers, are communication-driven with an IEP team proficient in child's communication mode; parents are included as equal partners.

Tips for Parents

Part C to B Transition

Transitions between early intervention and preschool services often create anxiety for parents due to the shift from family-focused to child-centered services. Further, the issues associated with hearing loss and the responsibility of making the right choices for their child's future often result in a time of uncertainty that is exacerbated by an education process that can seem unwelcoming.

There are a number of strategies that can minimize the concern for parents (Johnson, 2001).

1. *Prepare for the IFSP/IEP transition meeting.* Parents should visit preschools and meet with the preschool teachers and other staff prior to the transition meeting. It's often helpful for parents to bring along another parent or family member or the family's early intervention specialist so that there's someone with whom they can discuss their visit. The preschool teacher may also be willing to meet with family members in the home. Parents may also want to bring another person to support them at the transition meeting. Parents should be familiar with their rights as well as service obligations for their child under Part B of IDEA prior to the transition meeting.

2. *Think of preschool as transition.* Recognize that transition doesn't have to happen in six months. Think about the entire preschool experience as the transition between early intervention and school-age programs. This way the benefits of family-focused services can be combined with the language and social experiences of early education programs.

3. *Maintain consistent and effective communication.* Families need to feel that their input is valued and schools should listen carefully to what families are saying. Weekly written information and follow-up phone calls from the school help maintain open com-

munication. Parents should be encouraged to ask questions and seek clarification of information.

4. *Establish roles and expectations together.* Families need a game plan. They need to know what to expect from school as well as what's expected of them. Discuss this relationship with your child's school so that everyone is clear about respective roles and responsibilities.

5. *Continue home visits.* Home visiting is the hallmark of early intervention programs. Why should they end with the transition to Part B? Home visits give teachers and parents an opportunity to maintain consistent, effective communication. It also gives the teacher an opportunity to support and provide information to parents, to view the child in the familiar environment of the home, and to observe the communication styles used in the home.

6. *Have flexible programs and schedules.* Young children entering preschool for the first time may not be ready for the same preschool experience as that of older preschool children. Parents can discuss with the school the amount of time that their child will attend preschool. For some children, a combination of home-based support and preschool may be most effective.

7. *Use the Communication Plan.* The methodology biases of professionals have caused parents perhaps more consternation than any other aspect of raising and educating a child with hearing loss. It is communication not the method that's critical to the child's development. Families and school professionals should develop a Communication Plan to identify how the child communicates and determine how that communication will be accommodated and supported.

8. *Establish a parent support group.* Parents benefit from getting together to share and learn from one another's experiences. Elicit the help of a "seasoned" parent to assist the school to organize the support group and to plan activities. Childcare, carpooling

or other transportation options and snacks help with attendance. Establish a calling tree to communicate with parents and to remind them of events. Provide interpreters whenever possible to accommodate family members who are deaf or hard-of-hearing or non-English speaking families.

9. *Facilitate kindergarten visitations.* Begin kindergarten visitations in the winter and spring prior to entrance into kindergarten to develop rapport with the teacher and familiarity with the school and classroom. Be sure that the kindergarten teacher has all pertinent information and understands the child's IEP needs, goals and services.

[NOTE: In addition, the Appendix 5-D document, Preschool/ Kindergarten Placement Checklist for Children who are Deaf and Hard-of-Hearing, will aid parents and their early intervention provider in evaluating preschool options to assist in identifying the best preschool placement. This checklist, in an indirect way, establishes standards and expectations for sound educational programming.]

Getting Through the IEP

The IEP process is less intimidating when parents are knowledgeable about their rights and the provisions of IDEA. One of the most significant byproducts of early identification and intervention is that parents are more savvy and prepared to advocate for their child when they enter Part B services. Here are some pointers:

1. *Be Knowledgeable.* Review the special education laws and know your rights. Two excellent resources are *The Complete IEP Guide* (Siegel, 2000) and *Wright'slaw* (Wright & Wright, 1999). Be particularly mindful of aspects of the law that are important for children with hearing loss, especially the communication considerations and audiology, assistive technology, and parent counseling and training services provi-

sions. Be familiar with the IEP form that is used by your child's school. Remember that the IEP meeting must be scheduled at a mutually agreed upon time and often can accommodate the work schedules of both parents.

2. *Build a relationship with your child's school teachers and support staff.* The parent/professional partnership cannot be overemphasized. Working together is about relationships and the better it is, the more you're able to work together to solve problems and create the best program for your child.

3. *Be realistic about what your child knows and can do.* Schools respect parents who have a good understanding of their child's skills and realistic expectations. Talk with your child about school, his/her strengths and challenges, and goals. Together discuss how those challenges are best supported. At the same time, maintain high expectations. Remember that you know your child best.

4. *Review assessment information before the IEP meeting.* It's difficult to absorb new information at the same time as you're developing goals and a service plan for your child. Set up an appointment to review all assessment information with specialists who have conducted the testing prior to the IEP meeting.

5. *Visit school and know your child's teachers and key staff.* Parent requests are more credible when they've taken the time to visit their child's school and classroom and to meet and talk with teachers and staff who are involved with their child. Parents may use the Placement Considerations Checklist for Students who are Deaf and Hard-of-Hearing in Appendix 5-E to assess the appropriateness of current and proposed classroom placements.

6. *Maintain records.* Start a file and always keep copies of your rights as presented by your child's school, every document (including the IEP) that requires your signature, progress reports, and all other relevant papers you receive.

7. *Know the IEP goals.* Review current IEP goals and take a written, prioritized list of the goals you have for your child to your meeting. Make sure your child's goals are consistent with the state and district standards for all students. Make sure the goals are specific, measurable, include a timeline for achievement. Ask for the research or evidence that supports that the practices implemented with your child in fact have a track record of working.

8. *Consider bringing a friend or advocate to the IEP meeting.* When a meeting requires a difficult decision, or may be contentious, it is often helpful to have another person accompany you who can help review information presented as well as assist you with the analysis of the information to make decisions. Advocacy groups provide professional advocates and are available in most communities to assist parents with objective opinions regarding the information. These advocates also know the legal details.

9. *Expect accountability.* In addition to assessing progress on IEP goals, ask your child's IEP team for data that demonstrates annual progress in all academic areas. Remember, barring other learning problems, the expectation should be for your child to make one year's growth in one year's time. If this progress is not achieved, ask why not. Are services being provided as specified on the IEP? Is placement appropriate? Are the teachers and other staff appropriately qualified? Are they doing their job?

10. *Do not be intimidated.* If you are uncomfortable with the IEP meeting, the recommendations, or your ability to make decisions during the meeting, you can request that the meeting be rescheduled or continued at a later time. You also don't have to sign the IEP at the meeting. If you have any questions, it is recommended that you take the IEP home and read it carefully. IEP information is summarized from the meeting discussions and may not always be written as you remembered or intended. If you have questions, make

a list and take it to the meeting so they can be addressed.

Special education can be a challenging system to understand and negotiate. Decisions must always be determined by performance data with the child's abilities and current functioning at the forefront. Parent and teacher goals should also be based on the same standards and expectations as exist for hearing children. How each child arrives at their goals is individually determined reflecting how a child's needs are best met rather than a value that one way is better than another.

The parent's relationship with their early intervention and education providers is key to the establishment of this long-term association. Mutual trust is established when communication is open and consistent. This partnership is critical to achieve a positive outcome for the child. Schools cannot educate children alone. Parents must recognize that they are their child's best advocate.

Resources for Parents

The Appendixes contain protocols that have been suggested in this chapter and that can be used by parents in the IFSP and IEP processes. In addition, lists are available for state education agency offices responsible for special education services for each state by going onto the Internet and conducting your own search. The state education agency has the ultimate authority and responsibility in each state to assure that children in special education receive appropriate services as determined by IDEA.

Professional organizations (listed in Appendix 5-F) provide an excellent source of information and support for parents. In addition, many of the hearing aid and cochlear implant manufacturers specialize in children and have educational information for parents.

Access to information has grown dramatically with the ever-expanding Worldwide Web. The Web now provides immediate access to a plethora of information about hearing loss and its treatments and interventions. Caution is recommended as some of this information represents opinion rather than evidence-based practice. Professional advice should always be sought before making significant decisions based on information gleaned from the Web. Appendix 5-F provides contact information for some of the most common resources that parents often find useful.

References

Colorado Department of Education (1996). The IDEA and Section 504 placement process. From Planning and Preparing Quality Individualized Education Programs, Section I, p.6. Denver: Self.

Hands and Voices (2001). Making the Grade: Are you satisfied with your child's education? www.handsandvoiceds.org.

Johnson, C.D. (2001). Supporting Families in Transition between Early Interventon and School-Age Programs. www.handsandvoices.org.

Siegel, L. (2000). *The Complete IEP Guide: How to advocate for your special ed child.* Berkeley: NOLO.

Siegel, L. (2002). The educational and communication needs of deaf and hard of hearing children: A statement of principle on fundamental educational change. American Annals of the Deaf, 145,(2), 64-77.

United States Department of Education (1992). Deaf Students Education Services, Policy Guidance. Federal Register, 57, 211, October 30, 1992, 49274-49276.

Wright, P. and Write, P. (1999). *Wright'slaw: Special Education Law.* Hartfield, VA: Harbor House Law Press, Inc.

Appendix 5-A: Communication Plan
For Child/Student who is Deaf/Hard-of-Hearing*

The IEP team has considered each area listed below, and has not denied instructional opportunity based on the amount of the child's/student's residual hearing, the ability of the parent(s) to communicate, nor the child's/student's experience with other communication modes.

1.   The child's/student's primary communication mode is one or more of the following:
- aural, oral, speech-based
- American Sign Language
- English-based manual or sign system

Issues considered:
Action Plan, if any:

2.   The IEP team has considered the availability of deaf/hard of hearing adult role models and peer group of the child's/student's communication mode or language.

Issues considered:
Action Plan, if any:

3. An explanation of all educational options provided by the administrative unit and available for the child/student has been provided.

Issues considered:
Action Plan, if any:

4.   Teachers, interpreters, and other specialists delivering the communication plan to the child/student must have demonstrated proficiency in, and be able to accommodate for, the child's/student's primary communication mode or language.

Issues considered:
Action Plan, if any:

5.   The communication-accessible academic instruction, school services, and extracurricular activities the child/student will receive have been identified.

Issues considered:
Action Plan, if any:

*From the Colorado Department of Education, Exceptional Student Services Unit. Reprinted with permission.

Appendix 5-B: IFSP Communication Plan*

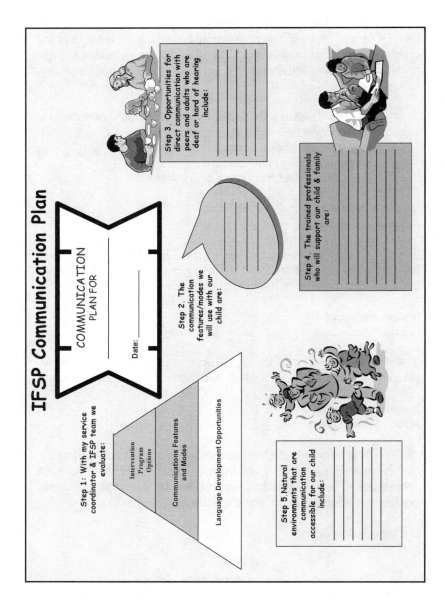

*From the Colorado Department of Education, Exceptional Student Services Unit. Reprinted with permission.

Appendix 5-C: IEP Checklist—Recommended Accommodations and Modifications For Students who are Deaf or Hard-of-Hearing*

Amplification Options

____ Personal hearing device (hearing aid, cochlear implant, tactile device)
____ Personal FM system (hearing aid + FM)
____ FM system/auditory trainer (without personal hearing aid)
____ Walkman-style FM system
____ Sound-field FM system

Assistive Devices

____ TDD
____ TV captioner
____ Other _____

Communication Accommodations

____ Specialized seating arrangements:_____
_____

____ Obtain student's attention prior to speaking
____ Reduce auditory distractions (background noise)
____ Reduce visual distractions
____ Enhance speechreading conditions (avoid hands in front of face, mustaches well-trimmed, no gum chewing)
____ Present information in simple, structured, sequential manner
____ Clearly enunciate speech
____ Allow extra time for processing information
____ Repeat or rephrase information when necessary
____ Frequently check for understanding
____ Educational interpreter (ASL, signed English, cued speech, oral)

Physical Environment Accommodations

____ Noise reduction (carpet & other sound absorption materials)
____ Specialized lighting
____ Room design modifications
____ Flashing fire alarm

(Continued on next page)

*From *Educational Audiology Handbook*, 1st edition by Johnson. Copyright 1997. Reprinted with permission of Delmar Learning, a division of Thomson Learning:www.thomsonrights.com.

(Appendix 5-C continued)

Instructional Accommodations

____ Use of visual supplements (overheads, chalkboard, charts, vocabulary lists, lecture outlines)
____ Captioning or scripts for television, videos, movies, filmstrips
____ Buddy system for notes, extra explanations/directions
____ Check for understanding of information
____ Down time/break from listening
____ Extra time to complete assignments
____ Step-by-step directions
____ Tutor
____ Note-taker

Curricular Modifications

____ Modify reading assignments (shorten length, adapt or elimi nate phonics assignments)
____ Modify written assignments (shorten length, adjust evaluation criteria)
____ Pre-tutor vocabulary
____ Provide supplemental materials to reinforce concepts
____ Provide extra practice
____ Alternative curriculum

Evaluation Modifications

____ Reduce quantity of tests
____ Use alternative tests
____ Provide reading assistance with tests
____ Allow extra time
____ Other modifications:_____

Other Needs/Considerations

____ Supplemental instruction (speech, language, pragmatic skills, auditory, speechreading skills)
____ Counseling
____ Sign language instruction
____ Vocational services
____ Family supports
____ Deaf/Hard of Hearing role models
____ Recreational/Social opportunities
____ Financial assistance
____ Transition services

Appendix 5-D: Preschool/Kindergarten Placement Checklist for Children who are Deaf and Hard of Hearing*

This checklist is intended to assist parents when considering preschool or kindergarten placement options for their deaf or hard of hearing child. The information should be obtained through observation and discussion with the current early intervention provider and the prospective teacher(s) and IEP team. Placement decisions should consider the child's communication, pre-academic, and social needs in the context of the proposed learning environment.

Teacher Interview

Name of School: _____   Date of Observation: _____

Individual Interviewed: _____
    Title: ___ Deaf Education Teacher   check type: ▢classroom   ▢itinerant ▢consultative
            ___ Preschool or Kindergarten Teacher   ___ Special Education Teacher   ___ Other
            If not a deaf education teacher/specialist, describe previous experience with children who   are deaf or hard of hearing:_____

Days program offered: _____   Hours per day: _____

Child's communication mode(s): _____   Mode(s) observed in classroom: _____

Total number of children in classroom: _____   Number of children with hearing loss: _____

Age span of children: ___ to ___   Child: adult ratio: ____

Average speaking/signing distance between teacher and child: ____ft

Number of children who are typical language models: ____

Amplification used or available: __Personal FM __Classroom FM/Infrared Other_____

Related and Support Services:

Area	Available?		Has had training with D/HH?		# of hours in classroom/week
Speech-language therapy	▢ Yes	▢ No	▢ Yes	▢ No	____
Educational audiology	▢ Yes	▢ No	▢ Yes	▢ No	____
Occupational therapy/physical therapy	▢ Yes	▢ No	▢ Yes	▢ No	____
Psychology	▢ Yes	▢ No	▢ Yes	▢ No	____
Counseling by psychologist or social worker	▢ Yes	▢ No	▢ Yes	▢ No	____

Other support services available: __Deaf/Hard of Hearing Role Models
    __Parent counseling and training   __Parent Support Groups/Activities
    __Transportation   __After school programs

Comments_____
_____
_____
_____

Classroom Observation

I. Classroom- Physical Environment   **YES**   **NO**

1. Is the room size conducive to learning? (A large room/high ceiling can distort sound; a small room may be noisier.)   ____   ____
2. Is the room adequately lit? (Lighting and shadows may affect speechreading and signing abilities.)   ____   ____
3. Is the ambient noise level for the classroom within recommended standards (noise ≤35dbA and reverberation ≤.6 msec, ANSI S12.60.2002)?   ____   ____
4. Is the room treated to reduce noise (carpet on floor, acoustical ceiling tiles, window

(Continued on next page)

Appendix 5-D (con't)

coverings, cork or other wall coverings)?

5. Are noise sources in the classroom minimized (e.g., fish tanks, ventilation/heater fans, computers)? ____ ____

6. Does noise from adjacent spaces (hallways, outside the building) spill over into classroom? ____ ____

Comments_____

II. General Learning Environment   YES   NO

7. Does teacher(s)/adult(s) use a variety of techniques to elicit positive behavior from children? ____ ____

8. Are there a variety of centers (fine motor, art, manipulatives, science, music, dramatic play, sensory, literacy)? ____ ____

9. Is there a schedule identifying daily routines? ____ ____

10. Is there a behavior management system that provides clear structure for the class and consistent rules? ____ ____

11. Does the curriculum standards-based including a variety of themes, topics, and children's literature? ____ ____

12. Does the teacher use lesson plans to guide daily activities? ____ ____

13. Are activities modified to meet a variety of children's needs? ____ ____

Comments_____

III.   Instructional Style   YES   NO

14.   Classroom Discourse and Language
   a.   Are the teacher(s) and other adults good language models for the children? ____ ____
   b.   Is language consistently accessible to the child? ____ ____
            (If sign is used, do all adults in the classroom consistently sign, including their communications with other adults?)
   c.   Are peer responses repeated? ____ ____
   d.   Is vocabulary and language expanded by an adult? ____ ____

15. Teacher's Speaking Skills
   a.   Is enunciation clear? ____ ____
   b.   Is rate appropriate? ____ ____
   c.   Is loudness appropriate? ____ ____
   d.   Is facial expression used to clarify the message? ____ ____
   e.   Are gestures used appropriately? ____ ____
   f.   Are teacher's (or other speaker's) lips available for speechreading? ____ ____
   g.   Is teacher's style animated? ____ ____
   h.   Is a buddy system available to provide additional assistance or clarification? ____ ____

16. Use of Visual Information
   a.   Are props or other visual materials used for stories and activities? ____ ____
   b.   Are appropriate attention-getting strategies utilized? ____ ____
   c.   Are fingerplays, action songs, and dramatic play used in circle time, story time, centers, etc ____ ____

17. Small Group/Circle Time
   a.   Are all children encouraged to share and participate? ____ ____
   b.   Does the teacher face children when speaking? ____ ____
   c.   Do the children face one another when speaking? ____ ____
   d.   Does the teacher lead group activities in an organized, but child-friendly manner? ____ ____

Appendix 5-D (con't)

    e. Is appropriate wait time utilized to encourage children to think and
        participate? _____ _____
    f. Are children seated within the teacher's "arc of arms"? _____ _____
    g. Does teacher obtain eye contact prior to and while speaking? _____ _____
    h. Is the FM microphone passed around to all speakers? _____ _____

18. Use of Sign   ___Not Applicable
    a. Is sign consistently used by all adults in the class? _____ _____
    b. Is sign consistently used by all children in the class? _____ _____
    c. Does the type of sign used in the classroom match the signs used by this
        child? _____ _____
    d. Is fingerspelling used? _____ _____
    e. Are gestures used appropriately? _____ _____
    f. Are there opportunities for parents and peers to learn to sign? _____ _____

19. Opportunities for Hands-on Experience
    a. Are a variety of materials available? _____ _____
        Check those used: _books   _visual props   _audio tapes   _video tapes
                            _objects for dramatic play   _manipulatives
    b. Are stories experienced in a variety of ways? _____ _____
    c. Are there field trips? _____ _____
    d. Are cooking experiences available? _____ _____
    e. Are art and sensory activities conducted? _____ _____

20. Amplification/Equipment   ___Not Applicable
    a. Are personal amplification (hearing aids/cochlear implant) and assistive devices
        (FM, infrared) checked at school each day? _____ _____
    b. Is amplification used consistently in all learning environments? _____ _____

Comments_____

Reflection

IV. Individual Child Considerations   YES   NO

21. Language Considerations/Abilities
Think about how your child communicates thoughts, ideas, and needs. Think about
how your child communicates and interacts with other children. Will your child's
communication needs be nurtured in this classroom environment? Does the child
have sufficient language abilities to benefit from instruction in the classroom? Will _____ _____
this child develop English language competency in this environment

22. Social Interactions
Think about how your child plays alone and in groups. Think about how your child
interacts with other children. Will your child's social needs be nurtured in this _____ _____
classroom environment? Will this child be encouraged to develop self-advocacy
skills?

23. Auditory Skills
Does your child attend well? Is your child able to listen in noise? Think about what
your child does when he/she cannot hear? Does your child take responsibility for _____ _____
his/her hearing aids? Will your child's auditory needs be supported in this classroom
environment? In the lunchroom and other school environments? Is the staff qualified
and able to support the child's auditory needs?

Comments_____

V. School Culture   YES   NO

24. Is there evidence that the school administration supports students with
      disabilities? _____ _____
25. Is the school/district administrator knowledgeable about hearing loss? _____ _____
26. Is the school committed to making the necessary accommodations for
      children with hearing loss? _____ _____
27. Is the teacher open to consultation with other professionals or specialists? _____ _____
28. Does the teacher provide opportunities for individualized attention? _____ _____
29. Is the teacher welcoming of children with special needs? _____ _____
30. Is the teacher willing to use amplification technology (hearing aids, FMs,
      cochlear   implants)? _____ _____

Comments_____

Appendix 5-E: Placement Considerations Checklist for Students who are Deaf and Hard-of-Hearing*

This checklist is intended to assist with placement considerations for deaf or hard of hearing students. Information should be obtained through observation and discussion among the teachers, school staff, and parents. Placement decisions consider the student's communication, academic, and social needs in the context of the proposed learning environment.

Teacher Interview

Name of School: _____   Date of Observation: _____

Individual Interviewed: _____
　　___ Deaf Education Teacher　　check type: □classroom　　□itinerant □consultative　　□co-teacher
　　___ General Education Teacher　　___ Special Education Teacher　　___ Other
　　　　If not a deaf education teacher, describe previous experience with students who are deaf or hard
　　　　of hearing:_____

Grade: _____   Student: adult ratio in classroom: ____

Student's communication mode(s): _____   Mode(s) observed in classroom: _____

Student's language level: Receptive_____   Expressive_____

Total number of students in classroom: _____   Number of students with hearing loss: _____

Average speaking/signing distance between teacher and student: ____ft

Amplification used or available: __Personal FM __Classroom FM/Infrared __None Other_____

Educational Interpreter assigned? __Yes __No   Meets state's minimum standard? __Yes __No

Related and Support Services:

Area	Available?		Has had training with D/HH?		# of hours in classroom/week
Speech-language therapy	□ Yes	□ No	□ Yes	□ No	____
Educational audiology	□ Yes	□ No	□ Yes	□ No	____
Occupational therapy/physical therapy	□ Yes	□ No	□ Yes	□ No	____
Psychology	□ Yes	□ No	□ Yes	□ No	____
Counseling by psychologist or social worker	□ Yes	□ No	□ Yes	□ No	____

Other support services available:　　　　　　　　　__Deaf/Hard of Hearing Role Models
__Parent counseling and training　　　　　　　　__Parent Support Groups/Activities
__Transportation　　　　　　　　　　　　　　　__After school programs

Comments_____
_____
_____

Classroom Observation

I. Classroom- Physical Environment	YES	NO
1. Is the room size conducive to learning? (A large room/high ceiling can distort sound; a small room may be noisier.)	____	____
2. Is the room adequately lit? (Lighting and shadows may affect speechreading and signing abilities.)	____	____
3. Is the ambient noise level for the classroom within recommended standards (noise ≤35dbA and reverberation ≤.6 sec, ANSI S12.60.2002)?	____	____

Appendix 5-F: Resources for Parents

Parent Organizations

American Society for Deaf Children
www.deafchildren.org
1-800-942-2732
717-334-7922 (TTY)

Hands and Voices
www.handsandvoices.org

Professional Organizations

Alexander Graham Bell Association for the Deaf and Hard of Hearing
www.agbell.org
1-866-337-5220
202-337-5221 (TTY)

American Academy of Audiology (AAA)
www.audiololgy.org
1-800-222-2336
703-790-8466 (TTY)

American Speech-Language-Hearing Association (ASHA)
www.asha.org 1-800-638-8255
301-897-5700 (TTY)

Auditory-Verbal International, Inc
www.auditory-verbal.org
703-739-1049
703-739-0874 (TTY)

Boys Town National Research Hospital
www.boystownhospital.org/parents/index.asp
555 N. 30th St.
Omaha, NE 68131

Educational Audiology Association
www.edaud.org
1-800-460-7EAA

Laurent Clerc National Deaf Education Center
www.clerccenter.gallaudet.edu/InfoToGo
202-651-5051 (V/TTY)

National Institute on Deafness and Other Communication
Disorders www.nidcd.nih.gov
1-800-241-1044
1-800-241-1055 (TTY)

Special Education and Legal Resources

National Association of State Directors of Special Education
www.nasdse.org

National Deaf Education Project
www.ndepnow.org

Wrights Law
www.wrightslaw.org

U. S. Department of Education, Office of Special Education
Programs
www.ed.gov/about/offices/list/osers

INDEX

A

B

C